Praise for **The Art of Trying**

"Benita relays the all-important narrative of the reality of infertility. It is not simply a physical experience, more something that envelops your entire essence of being. Her raw honesty and gentle advice will undoubtedly bring comfort to many, many women."

– Lucy Coffin, Registered Nurse & Fertility Therapist

"Benita takes the reader on a reproductive journey. It is an emotional and very open account experienced by many women. As health professionals, we only see a small part of the struggle. I feel privileged to have been on this journey and gained a new found respect and understanding of couples having difficulty conceiving. Well done Benita!"

– Dr. Anna Carswell, GP Obstetrician & Medical Educator

"So much more than a book for those trying to conceive!

Anything that wasn't urgent went out the window for a couple of days because I couldn't put the book down! The challenges I have faced are very different than Benita's, but her story is so enlightening and interesting on so many levels – really a book that anyone, male or female, could pick up and get so much from.

So many of us know how it feels when our bodies feel out of control due to a health issue. Or when the plans we have for our life just don't work out. The Art of Trying is a book about never giving up.

I am so grateful that through Benita's story I have a greater awareness and sensitivity for those trying to conceive. It is a compelling reminder to always be kind and thoughtful with the topics of fertility, pregnancy and mental health. You really never know what someone may be going through – books like this are vital in starting and continuing dialogue and awareness of the struggles of so many.

A real stand out of this book is the beautiful kindness and love Benita shows her readers as she bravely and generously shares her personal journey in the hope that it will make their path a little easier."

– Susan Hatchett, Artist, Graphic Designer & Mother

"Benita shares her story in a practical and heartfelt way to help others, and it has given me the opportunity to experience IVF from the other side of the desk."

– Dr. Mark Livingstone, Fertility & IVF Specialist

"There is more to this book than just one couple's fascinating conception journey told with genuine warmth, spirit and naked honesty. Benita's passion and sincerity comes through to the reader; you are there with her – on the tractor, or at the kitchen bench at the farm, as she brings you along to shed light on subjects that are too often kept in the dark.

Anyone who is struggling, or has struggled, with infertility will find solace and solidarity in this story. Anyone who is supporting someone else's struggles will benefit enormously from better understanding the raw, complex road that they face. But this book offers more than just insight; it is an enlightening, entertaining and engaging read that dives into a world that looks similar and yet is quite distant from our own."

– Mandy, Mother & Consumer Insights Researcher

"There is no battle more painful, private and lonely than that of the road to conception. Especially when you are isolated either geographically or by the unspeakably cruel circumstances of being 'the only woman left on the shelf' without little people to call your own. As somebody who walked that road and never could have my own family, I cannot stress enough the devastating impact this can have on a woman's mind, body and soul. It can crush you to pieces and leave you wondering if there is anything left to hope for. It strips you to your bare bones and leaves you feeling lost, utterly. Women need to be far better equipped for the challenges of this walk and the potential mental health ramifications that still aren't discussed with enough weight.

I absolutely take my hat off to Benita for tackling this topic, front on."

– Shanna Whan, Rural Personality & Founder of Sober in the Country

"An enjoyable, informative read that shares the highs and lows one couple endured to achieve their dream of becoming parents while living in rural Australia. I couldn't put it down!"

– Jo, Mother, Business Owner & Photographer

the art of trying

An intimate account of my journey to conceive

| WITH ORIGINAL JOURNAL ENTRIES |

Benita Bensch

Editor: Corinne Casazza
corinnecasazza@gmail.com

Cover & Book Design: Anne Karklins
anne@hasmarkpublishing.com

Cover Photo: Jo Shanahan Photography

Author Photo: Hannah McNulty, Dalli Photography

ISBN 13: 978-1-989161-94-4

ISBN 10: 1989161944

Hasmark
PUBLISHING

This book is dedicated to

All the women in the trying club who know what I mean

and

Adam, who has sustained me – before, during and after the trying.

TABLE OF CONTENTS

PREFACE

Trying, short for 'trying to conceive' (TTC), is a colloquial term commonly used to describe the process of deliberately timing intercourse to coincide with ovulation for the purpose of creating an embryo.

When used in this context the word 'trying' implies action, however it's 'try' that's the action word – the verb. 'Trying' is not, it's a descriptive word – an adjective. Here is a definition:

> **trying** /ˈtrʌɪɪŋ/ adj. annoying; distressing; irritating; testing one's patience. – *Macquarie Dictionary*

According to this, 'trying' is a highly fitting word to describe how I felt the majority of the time that I was TTC. I came to detest the word because it invoked in me a sense of hard work, futility and never quite getting there. What got to me about TTC was that it was the one thing in my life in which the degree of trying was not directly correlated to results. Trying a lot could work, or we might get the result effortlessly despite the trying, not because of it.

The Art of Trying is my very personal story of TTC stemming from my journal entries from 2010 to 2017. The title arose organically because achieving conception felt like a rare and complex art form to me, whereby everything had to come together in perfect alignment.

My story is not especially extraordinary. I am not a celebrity; I don't have an against-all-odds infertility story, and so many women have been through far worse than me. For many years that held me back from sharing my story. I didn't feel like it was bad enough. I didn't feel worthy. But the niggling feeling to document what I had experienced wouldn't go away. I believe that in life we are called to do things that we don't necessarily understand at the time, but if only we will have the courage to listen to our inner knowing, we will come to understand.

So, I kept writing a little at a time, even though I wasn't sure what the end purpose was, and the fear and doubt kept trying to block me. Initially, I didn't know if I was writing this book for me or for others. Time has shown me that it's both. Writing *The Art of Trying* has been incredibly healing for me. It is told from my heart and I have cried many tears throughout its creation. I have had to retrace my steps, revisit my records and relive all the memories and feelings from those years to get to this point.

Just when I'd think about letting go of the idea of this book, I'd find myself in another conversation with a woman having TTC challenges. And it would spur me on, that if my story could help just one person to feel more supported and know "it's not just me" then it would be worth it. That's what *I* wanted, what I *needed*, when we were TCC – real stories written by real people, so that I would feel... less alone. It was a terribly isolating time going through infertility in the bush.

The Art of Trying is uniquely my story but across the world it's a shared story with common threads. So, while writing, I kept in my heart and mind the friends who have:

- Been trying to conceive since we started, with no success
- Had one baby through the help of IVF but never succeeded in having another
- Never been able to conceive, full stop
- Birthed two children with ease then experienced secondary infertility
- Polycystic ovary syndrome going through IVF
- Birthed one child and then only miscarriages

These are but a few heartbreaking stories from the masses. Infertility does not discriminate. Their stories are not mine to tell, but I hope that through my words, I can somehow honour their pain and their courage.

The Art of Trying is not a how-to book. If you're looking for fertility or medical advice on how to get pregnant, you won't find it here. What you *will* find is an open, candid and detailed account of the dark and the light I experienced while TTC at different times over seven years. *The Art of Trying* explores some painful topics that I hope will help shape different perceptions and start new conversations around TTC.

Before you begin reading, I'd like to make special mention of my husband Adam, who you will meet in the first chapter, and get to know throughout the book. From the outset Adam made it clear that this should be my story and that he didn't wish to contribute directly. The way I see it *The Art of Trying* is very much *our* story told from *my* perspective. He is a very integral part of it and TTC impacted him as much as it did me, just in a different way. I commend him for his bravery to indirectly open up about this difficult topic, and for allowing me to share intimate details from our private life. He is an incredible man and I am privileged to share my life with him.

The Art of Trying is for anyone who needs it. I hope it meets you where you're at on your journey, and that it cradles you in your time of need. With my blessing, you can choose the sections that resonate with you and take from it what you're seeking. My wish is that my story also helps the families and friends of those who are TTC to better understand, and better support them.

HOW TO USE THIS BOOK

The Art of Trying is made up of three main components:

1. The narrative
2. Journal entries
3. Special notes

I have written this book in such a way that you could read the narrative alone and take away the bulk of the main story. But you will gain a much deeper insight into my experience and live it through my eyes by reading the journal entries as well. The narrative is written retrospectively, whereas the journal entries give a precise snapshot of what I was doing, thinking and feeling at that particular point in time. There is also important detail within the journal entries not re-told elsewhere.

The special notes are additional but complementary to the narrative. In these sections I explore and reflect on significant topics arising from my experiences.

Chapter 13 written by guest author Karen Brook, and Chapter 14 – *Affirmations*, are bonus chapters to aid you in developing a positive mindset conducive to conceiving.

In the final pages, you'll find an Appendix which includes a list of abbreviations, a summary of the medical results from our assisted reproductive technology treatments, and resources for your use.

Medical disclaimer
This is my personal journey of TTC. It is in no way intended to be a substitute for professional medical advice. Please contact a qualified medical professional for advice and treatment.

CHAPTER 1

Trying not to try...
but actually trying a little

The sound of the contraceptive pill packet hitting the bottom of the waste bin in our Fiji honeymoon suite was music to my ears. I tossed it in there with such jubilation that I felt I might burst. I was free! Free from the self-imposed chains of the pill that had impacted the natural rhythm of my body for 12 years. And free from the barrier that had protected me from becoming a mother all that time. This was historic. FINALLY we were married. FINALLY we were going to start a family!

I have always wanted children. Actually, that's a little bit of a lie because come to think of it, when I was young I wanted to live in a shed with only my horses, cattle and dogs (and probably guinea pigs) and never get married. I can't be sure when, but I transitioned out of that phase at some point.

Apart from the crazy shed lady phase, I never questioned *if* I would have children, only when, how many, and with whom. As a young woman I considered 27 to be the perfect age to start breeding (not too young, not too old) and a tribe of four seemed like the perfect number. If all went well, I'd be done and dusted with child bearing a smidge past 30. I probably have a written goal for it somewhere.

Goals have always been my thing. People who know me well would describe me as ambitious and a high achiever. It came naturally from an early age to repeatedly find my growth edge and go beyond it, to be the best I can, to take opportunities, or even better – create them. As a little girl it wasn't enough for me to have a few guinea pigs as pets. I started my first business breeding and selling them to the pet shop, and then wrote a book (which I still treasure) about them, complete with photographs and hand-drawn illustrations. During lunch breaks I would type up the pages on the only computer I had access to at the small state primary school I attended. I didn't know it at the time, but before I turned 10, I achieved my first life goal of starting a business.

In my senior years at Murgon State High School it wasn't enough to be a school captain, I was also president of the student council, captain of our sporting house, awarded equal dux of our school, rotary student of the year, and best and fairest of our women's soccer team.

In my third year of University in 2001 I fulfilled my goal to complete a six month student exchange to Purdue University in Indiana. I'd never stepped foot on an aircraft until the morning I boarded the 14 hour flight in Brisbane bound for Los Angeles, on my own. I was so anxious that I barely slept the night before, or on the flight, but I did it.

You get the picture. I am always on a mission and at my best when I'm contributing, growing and working on a project. I'm entrepreneurial. 'Bored' has never entered my vocabulary; to the contrary – I have always wanted to fit more into a day and my life than is physically possible. I want to embrace *everything*.

I wasn't very maternal once upon a time. I could attend a baby shower or children's birthday party and not touch a little person. I didn't like babysitting. I was happy to be around children but I never had that *love* for them that some women have. "I just love kids," they'd squeal and I would think, "but why!?" However, I knew it would feel different with my own, and I presumed marriage and children (in that order thank you very much) would be in my future.

Boys. I've loved them for as long as I can remember. Love letters, scribbled hearts and initials on my pencil case, catch-and-kiss behind the primary school toilet block, dreamy pages dedicated to them in my diary, smooches on the trampoline… boys were also my thing. Ask my Mum; she'll tell you I always had a boyfriend (or two!) on the go and it was always very serious love. Poor Mum, I feel for her that she's had to live through the ups and downs of my love affairs over the years. I never spent a moment daydreaming about a big white wedding, but I often wondered about the man out there in the universe who would one day become my life partner.

I knew love a few times as I morphed into adulthood, but I didn't know the extent of love until I met Adam in May 2005, a month shy of my 24th birthday.

I was having a quiet drink with my friend Lucy at a pub in Armidale, New South Wales (NSW) when I spotted a tall, handsome young man looking over from the next room. I'd never seen him before. Who was that? He and Lucy had met before, which is what drew his attention in the first place. It wasn't until we were at the next pub up the street (our mutual favourite it turned out) that he approached us at the bar.

"Who's your friend?" he asked Lucy, giving me a charming grin.

"Hi, I'm Benita." I was unsure of what I thought of this young buck, and wary he was going to try a pick up line on me.

The few beers under his belt gave him more confidence than he actually had, evident only because I was stone cold sober. I was completing a graduate diploma in business studies and had an assignment due in two days that I hadn't started, so I was forcing myself to behave that night.

"G'day I'm Adam Bensch," he said, hand outstretched, still with that grin.

"Bench as in bench, like sitting on the bench?" I questioned with a mixture of curiosity and cheekiness, as I shook his big, warm bear paw.

"No, Bensch with a silent "s" actually," he said with a sincerity that told me he was proud of his name and it wasn't the first time he'd answered that question.

"Where are you from?" I asked.

"Grong Grong," He said.

"Grong what!?" I'd never heard of it.

This just kept getting better. Adam Bensch from Grong Grong. Who was this guy and why had I never met him? There was a something about him that had me curious. We chatted a little longer, he was impressed that I was drinking a XXXX Gold stubbie, and we made a bet about who would win the State of Origin rugby league match the following week (he is from NSW, I'm from Queensland). There was some flirting, but I was still deciding if I wanted him to stay or leave Lucy and I alone. His mates were goading him from down the bar and he soon went back to them.

The events of the evening resulted in me – still sober – driving Adam's mates, Lucy and Adam (in the boot of the car) back to their house in my silver Ford Falcon sedan. He wooed me with heavy metal music in his bedroom and talked non-stop. After a few hours I *really* had to get home to bed, but not without him giving me his number, and the exchange of a sneaky moonlight kiss on the way to my car. Damn it felt good. I was a goner.

We'd both lived in Armidale at the same time for three years, and even overlapped one year of studying the same Rural Science degree, yet we'd never met. It was Adam's fourth year of University when we did meet, which is a good thing as I might not have liked younger, wilder Adam as much. He was about to turn 22, was still enjoying the delights that Uni living has to offer, and not at all interested in a serious relationship. I was in my third year of work at the Agricultural Business Research Institute and had plans to leave town before Christmas, so nurturing our courtship didn't make much sense.

Sometimes things in life don't make sense, but we do them anyway. I knew I was setting myself up for hurt, but couldn't stay away from this character who had stolen my heart. It didn't make sense either to stay together when Adam moved to Canada after Uni and I moved back to Queensland (Qld), but we remained in close contact. There was something special between us that neither of us could ignore.

Our relationship was non-committal and leisurely to evolve, but strengthened and deepened steadily over the next few years. It was tested by the challenges of distance, but at its core bolstered by our shared values, our love for one another and mutual love for agriculture. We moved in together and set up our first home in November 2007.

Everyone loves "Benschy" when they meet him. It's hard not to. He's good-natured, patient, kind, generous, easy going, loving, hard-working, funny, clever and ambitious. He's a man of great integrity and morals and a natural at most things he tries his hand at (although he would never admit it). A social bloke; you might say a 'typical' country boy who loves his farming, rugby and a beer. He is tall, broad and handsome, with black (now greying) curly hair and a cheeky smile. Put simply – he's a loveable, top bloke, from a salt-of-the-earth farming family.

He and I grew up 1,200 kilometres apart, but there were many simi-larities between our upbringings. A mother, father and siblings, farming, school, sport and an occasional holiday to the beach are things we had in common. I have a brother Shawn and two sisters Kylee and Terri, while

Adam comes from a family of three boys, within an extended family of many boys. There are a lot of Bensch men! Girl stuff was most certainly not on his radar when he met me, and I think he would have gladly kept it that way if he had a choice. Initially he cringed and squirmed uncomfortably at the mention of the monthly 'p' word. Boy, was he in for a shock hanging with me, poor guy, as he gradually came to know the challenges I had with heavy, painful periods, erratic bleeding, and the numerous methods of attempting to manage this.

Adam was in no rush to get married, bless him. I, on the other hand, was impatient by the time he proposed to me on one knee on top of Mount Kaputar in March 2010. I even considered proposing to him for fear he was never going to ask me. I doubt that would have gone down well. In true Adam style, the more I hinted/nagged, the longer he took, so I had to wait until he was good and ready. My patience wasn't tested because I was unsure of his commitment to me, but because I could hear the resounding thud of my biological clock ticking. I was not far off turning 29. We were lagging – in my grand plan there was supposed to be a baby by now!

Tick, tick, tick.

We were wed near Gunnedah in a beautiful country garden ceremony followed by a marquee reception on the sixteenth of October 2010. Surrounded by a hundred of our family and friends, I made this promise to Adam:

Adam, all that I am and all that I have,
I offer you today and from this day forward.
You are my best friend, the love of my life, and
I choose you as my husband above all others.
I promise to encourage and inspire you, to laugh with you, and
to comfort you in times of sorrow and struggle.
I promise to love you in good times and in bad,
to always accept you as you are and to be forever faithful.
I promise to cherish you, respect and honour you, and,
for you, be the most that I can.
As we grow together, I will walk with you wherever life may lead us
and whatever may come.
These things I give to you today, and all the days of our life.

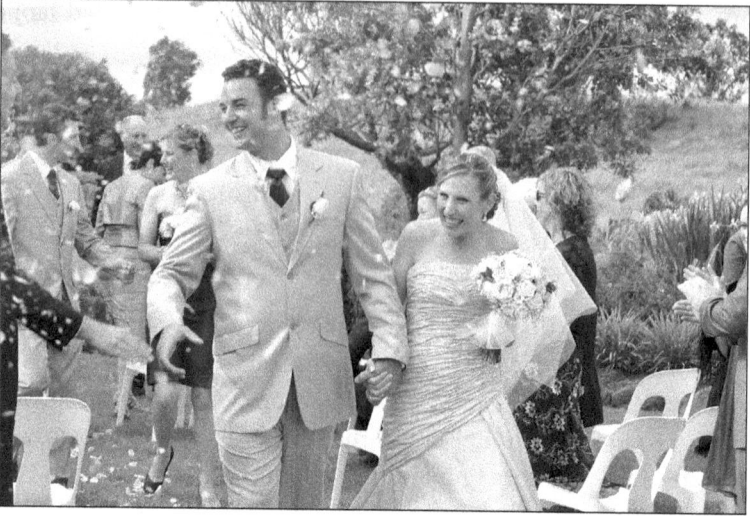

The glorious day we said "I do" and I became Mrs Bensch, Gunnedah October 2010.

Off we flew to Fiji a few days later.

FINALLY the pill was in the bin and I was going to join the Trying to Conceive (TTC) aka 'trying' club... even if it was a few years later than I had envisaged. But hold up, not yet, as I was advised by my gynaecologist to hold off trying for a few months after stopping the pill – to get it out of my system. Agh, I didn't want more waiting, I wanted to make babies! But I did what I was told. I thought I was so in control during those months, almost martyr-like, with a secret that no one else knew: we were going to start trying!

I was so envious of my friends who had stopped taking the pill up to 12 months before they started trying. Why didn't I go off the pill earlier in readiness too, you ask? Because I used the pill to help manage the condition I have: endometriosis. With endometriosis, when you menstruate, the uterine-like cells that have developed in other parts of your reproductive tract still behave like uterine cells, and shed blood into areas they shouldn't, which creates scar tissue. This can cause problems with conception, and other things. So, I used a contraceptive to suppress the build-up of scar tissue. For me, the best scenario was either to be on the pill or pregnant!

My gynaecologist suggested that endometriosis *may* impact conceiving a child but since my Mum and older sister Kylee had no trouble falling pregnant, I should be fine, and not to worry. I had heard many times how both could get pregnant as easily as looking at their husbands. I hoped it would be the case for me too, but based on my less-than-straightforward gynaecological history, I had a lurking feeling that starting a family would continue in the same vein.

We 'officially' started trying in December 2010. Despite growing up on a farm and being well aware of the coming-together of a male and female needing to be well-timed, I was hilariously oblivious about what that meant for us humans. I had no idea about ovulation, when or even if, I ovulated! What struck me was how small the conception window is. My thoughts: how the bloody hell does *anyone* get pregnant!?

I took a rough guess as to when our window was – challenging as my cycle was wobbling all over the place. I hadn't had a regular period in a long time and I had been on so many hormonal concoctions over the years that my body needed to detox and find its natural cadence again. I felt like there was no time for that.

During those precious early months of trying, I was attempting to play it cool, trying not to think about it too much, pretending as if we weren't really trying, like it was going to magically happen for us. I wanted us to be one of those freakish couples that conceive in their first month without even meaning to (you know the ones).

Whilst I had been forewarning Adam (and myself) for a few years that it could take a while to conceive, that didn't seem to stop me from setting my early expectations WAY too high. For whatever crazy reason (practising positive thinking probably), I was hopeful I'd be pregnant around the end of the year and subsequently only narrowly miss the goalpost of having a baby by age 30.

I told myself not to expect to fall pregnant, but inevitably my hopes escalated towards the end of each cycle and were then dashed as my period arrived. The end of the year came and went. I placated myself with "it's still early days, Benita."

The start of trying resulted in an instant change in mindset for me around intercourse. I would go so far as to say that it was never the same again. Previously, it had been purely for pleasure. Now we were in foreign territory. Intercourse had a new purpose, an end goal, and that introduced a swag of thoughts and feelings with it. It really heralded a new chapter in my life, and in our relationship.

My frustration began as the months went on without triumph. And the research scientist in me emerged. How could I help this process along?

A special note on Endometriosis

Endo-what? That's what I thought too when I properly paid attention to the word for the first time – in a groggy, partially incoherent state waking from the general anaesthetic in February 2007. "We did find endometriosis," my Doctor said. "We'll talk about it when I see you in a few weeks."

Endometriosis is a condition where tissue similar to the endometrium, which normally lines the uterus, is found at sites outside the uterus – most often in the pelvis and lower abdomen. These deposits can cause a number of problems such as pelvic pain and infertility, though it is possible you can have endometriosis and not experience either. Endometriosis is sneaky, as the degree of the problem does not always indicate the damage the disease is causing.

My experience with endometriosis began many years before I became aware of it. As a teenager and young adult it was the norm for me to have heavy bleeding and long, painful periods. It was a time of the month I truly dreaded. I vividly recall lying on the couch for most of one particular Christmas day because I was in too much pain to participate in the festivities. And there were plenty of those occasions. I used anti-inflammatory tablets, heat packs and movement to relieve the symptoms. I knew not everyone's periods were like mine, but thought that's just how it was for me and didn't question it. I got a little relief once I started to take the contraceptive pill at age 17.

As a 24-25-year-old woman in 2005/6, I had an annoying problem with almost continual breakthrough bleeding in the second half of my cycle. It went on for about 18 months and was really affecting my self-confidence and intimacy, so I eventually went to see a local female general practitioner (GP) about it. I had no idea what could be done, but I knew the bleeding wasn't normal, and it was impacting my life enough that it was time to take action.

This GP's reaction shocked and upset me so much that it's forever burned in my memory. She essentially dismissed my concerns and told me there was nothing wrong; that it was just the way my body was. In a nutshell – put up with it. I implored her that something wasn't right and surely I didn't have to put up with it. It took all my resolve not to cry or yell.

As calmly and assertively as I could, I asked her to write me a referral to see a gynaecologist whose name I had with me. She was not too pleased about me wanting to go around or above her, but I held my ground until she gave me the referral. Thank goodness I did.

Fast forward to February 2007. After trying to control the bleeding via numerous contraceptive pills without success, my gynaecologist and I decided on a hysteroscopy and laparoscopy to check out what was going on inside my reproductive tract. The possibility of endometriosis was mentioned, but we didn't jump to surgical treatment right away because I didn't have the full gamut of classic endometriosis symptoms like pain during intercourse or unexplained chronic pelvic pain. I tried first line management and that failed, so surgical management was the next step.

Also thrown in the mix was a lesion on my cervix that hung around for a few years, requiring treatment and monitoring with what felt like 500 pap smears. Surgery provided the opportunity to cauterise the lesion, so it seemed like a smart move. I was tired of the ongoing menstrual circus and wanted to know more about what was going on, so I was happy for the next step.

Laparoscopy is a surgical procedure performed under general anaesthetic where a small telescope is placed through a hole made at your belly button, allowing the surgeon to see and assess the organs of the pelvis and abdomen. Two other holes were made further out either side of my abdomen to assist with the laparoscope. The laparoscopy magnifies the endometrium-like tissues and even small amounts of disease can be seen. Tissue that is thought to contain endometriosis is destroyed or removed, and sent to pathology to confirm the diagnosis. At the same time, I had the hysteroscopy to examine the inside of my uterus.

I was diagnosed with mild to moderate endometriosis. This was a shock, and also a relief, because it provided me with a diagnosis to work with. My philosophy is that it's always better to know. The patches of endometriosis were destroyed using diathermy during the procedure (see Appendix for locations). In the years that followed I continued on a merry-go-round of different contraceptive pills and the Depo Provera® needle (which I had an allergic reaction to every time) to prevent me from having a period so the endometrial cells wouldn't build up again. That ride is a story in itself and it took me up until the pill packet got thrown in the bin on our honeymoon.

Countless women suffer much more heavily at the hand of endometriosis than I have. Awareness and understanding of the disease are increasing but for how common it is endometriosis is still largely hidden in the shadows and its victims suffer in silence. These are the women who call in sick for the day, but are embarrassed to explain why. The women who soldier on crippled-over with chronic pain for years because no one can tell them the cause; the young women at high school desperately praying that when they stand up they won't have a flood of blood that soaks through their skirt. The women trying for a baby and wondering why they aren't falling pregnant. They are everywhere.

Don't let anyone tell you differently to what you know to be true about your body! If something feels wrong, it probably is. You know your body better than anyone. Trust your inner voice. Follow up on anything unusual and be a strong advocate for your own health. Become informed, ask questions and seek a second opinion if you're not happy with the outcome of a medical consultation. You don't have to put up with debilitating pain and problems that affect your everyday life. It's your body and your life. When it comes to your health, and particularly reproductive health, don't delay your investigations.

CHAPTER 2

Trying a lot

As the months of 'trying a little' started to roll one into the next, the lurking little voice in my head that said: "I knew it... I knew this wouldn't happen easily for us," grew louder. Really, I was jumping the gun; it's normal for it to take a while for the average couple to conceive. As I was under 35, I had been advised that we should try naturally for at least a year before seeking assistance, so that's the guideline I was adhering to. There was always a tug-of-war raging within me – not wanting to overreact, but not leave things too long either, just in case we did end up needing help to create a baby.

Me being me, wanting to do everything in my power to make this thing happen, I started to do the things trying people do when they really want a baby, beginning with charting my basal body temperature. Apparently, our basal body temperature drops just before ovulation and then rises suddenly afterwards, so by taking and recording temperature every day over a period of a few months, a pattern should emerge as to when the most fertile period is. At this stage my cycle length was still ranging between 32 and 43 days, so my goal was to pinpoint, or at least narrow down, the elusive fertile period.

I bought the special basal body temperature thermometer from the pharmacy that comes with a graph on a piece of paper, onto which you plot your temperature every day (hint: it helps to photocopy this piece of paper a few times before you write on it so that you have a blank chart for subsequent months). Each morning in bed before you do anything that might raise your temperature (e.g. eating, drinking, going to the toilet), you place the end of the thermometer under your tongue until you hear it beep. This activity should occur at the same time each day. There was definitely no temperature-raising trying practise allowed before my daily rendezvous with the thermometer. I was so paranoid about following the right procedure I'd hardly move a muscle in the process of reaching over to retrieve the thermometer from my bedside table.

I persevered with this for a few months and at one point excitedly thought I was onto some sort of trend, but in the end my graphs were up and down with no clear pattern. The whole thing messed with my head. Ultimately, this method was not well-aligned with my analytical, perfectionist tendencies because there were too many variables and I became stressed if I missed a day or didn't take my temperature at exactly the same time each day. Was I even doing it right? It also meant that TTC was first and foremost in my mind every morning which set me up for a few hours of thinking about it at the start of each day – a sure-fire way for it to grow into more of an obsession than it was already becoming.

Next up was observing my cervical mucus throughout the month. So subjective. A bit gross. More analysing. Is that watery and wet mucus? Or egg white and stretchy mucus? I had been making detailed notes about my cycle since going off the pill and had occasionally written things down like 'milky liquid' and 'chalky white' but the fertile mucus was never obvious to me. I wasn't at all confident in my deductions. Again, was I even doing it right? Even after years I was never able to rely upon mucus as a reliable indicator of my fertility. Kudos to those who can.

Ask a handful of women about what to do to optimise conception and they will all tell you something different. Each one will have their own theory on the best time of the month, how often to have sex, the best sexual position and likely also their own little special trick. For example: I have a friend who swore by having intercourse every day for five days in the middle of the month to fall pregnant (her body operated like clockwork with a regular 28 day cycle, mind you). Worked for her. And another friend who would lie with her legs in the air for 20 minutes after intercourse so 'it would all stay in there' while her husband brought her an orange juice. On reflection it's quite humorous what I learned about people's varying theories on optimising conception. I was no exception – we put plenty of them to the test.

Some months we were very committed to getting everything as 'right' as we possibly could, and other months our approach was more casual. Usually it depended on what else was going on at the time. As I was unsure when I ovulated, we aimed for intercourse every three days throughout the whole month with more frequency loosely around the middle of the month. I truly will never know what theories work or help, but what I know with 100% certainty is that you have to have sex to get pregnant. And sometimes a lot of it. Sounds obvious, I know. When you're in the trying-a-lot phase, it takes commitment and effort from both parties to keep up the act month after month. And the enthusiasm. Sex felt mechanical and obligatory at times… more than I cared to admit. I really disliked that. It wasn't helped by the fact that my mind was filled with thoughts like:

"I wonder if this will be *the* time."

"Oh gosh, what if this is *the* time?"

"I wonder if we should have had sex yesterday instead."

"Maybe we should be in a different position."

"If I orgasm will that increase our chances?"

It was hard to simply enjoy sex for what it was anymore.

Outside of TTC, at this point in time we were living in a rented farm-house on a property between Gunnedah and Tamworth in North West NSW. Adam was working as an Agronomist for a local company and I was very focused on building Sunburnt Country Consulting – my boutique marketing, media and events agency. It was in a growth stage and evolving rapidly with new projects, new team members and setting up a rented office space in Gunnedah. I was feeling the pressure that growth brings, but excited about the possibilities. I was fortunate to work with some beautiful, talented women in a similar stage of life and my vision was that the team would be equipped enough to keep the business running while I went part-time when our baby arrived. In the meantime, the bottom line of the business was my duty and I learned some tough lessons along the way. I loved my team and our work, but I found people management stressful. I was also transitioning from working solo at home to being a 'real' business owner with real responsibilities like business systems, wages, regular over-heads, bigger clients, a server, training, more marketing, delegating client work to my team and taking on more management work myself.

Trying a lot was gradually consisting of more and more theories, charting and analysing. With his beautiful good nature Adam was supporting me and going along with whatever I suggested we needed to do (he wasn't exactly doing any research at his end). Next I decided it was time to start using ovulation tests.

Ahhh yes, the good old ovulation test. It helps identify the two days of the month when you're most likely to get pregnant, by detecting the increase in luteinising hormone (LH) levels in urine that occurs 24-36 hours preceding ovulation. So basically you pee in a little cup at the same time each day (preferably in the afternoon, definitely not when you wake up – heaven forbid – oh, and try to reduce your liquid intake for two hours leading up to this) around the middle of the month, dip in the little strip that comes with the kit, wait for a line to appear (if you're lucky) and hope that it's a dark one to signal the surge in LH.

On the afternoons I was working at the Sunburnt Country office, I'd slink off to the downstairs toilet with my ovulation kit in hand, all the while anticipating if I was getting the timing right that month, had I drank too much fluid that day to dilute the test, and would today be *the* day? I imagined announcing to Adam on my arrival home that today was in fact *the* day and we would make passionate child-producing love, just like in the movies. Keep dreaming Benita. With more good humour than I was feeling, I'd sometimes share the shitty test result with 'the girls' (that I worked with) on my way back through the office. I didn't get one convincing dark line during the months that I used ovulation tests. It was another head fuck that left me wondering and anxious.

Of course, the general health of you and your partner has an important role to play in conceiving a baby and I had been diligently reading about the shoulds and should-nots when TTC.

Take a folic acid supplement. Tick! That one's easy.

Have a health check and blood tests prior to TTC. Tick! All clear.

Do not smoke or take drugs. Tick! Not my style.

Eat nutritious, healthy food. Tick! Mostly. Even gave fertility-friendly foods a go.

Do not be overweight. Tick! I was a svelte 63kg.

Limit caffeine. Tick! Neither of us drank coffee, didn't drink enough tea for it to be an issue and were sensible about things like chocolate and energy drinks.

Maintain regular exercise. Tick! Adam was playing rugby, I was playing soccer and we played touch football in the off season, as well as both exercising at home.

Avoid, or limit alcohol. We may have fallen down here. We were more conscious of our intake than ever before, and by no means heavy drinkers, but we enjoyed an alcoholic beverage or two in the evenings a few days a week. We liked to have a drink at weekend events with the occasional binge on rum and cola. I debated heavily on an ongoing basis whether I should be cutting out alcohol completely and demanding that Adam cut back. Would it really make that much difference? Surely the amount we drank wasn't a problem? I don't know. I did know myself well enough (or to be accurate – Adam knew me well enough!) to know that depriving myself of this small pleasure in life would cause me to focus on TTC even further – something I did not want.

Keep stress levels to a minimum. Hmmm perhaps a fail on my behalf here as I was feeling pretty stressed in my business, but I did my best to manage it.

Overall, I think we were in good health and there was nothing glaringly obvious that I perceived would dramatically impede our conception chances.

Since my late teens I have been a believer in the benefits of complementary therapies such as acupuncture, massage and naturopathy. About eight months into our official trying journey I went to see a herbalist about 150km away – Jenny – who came highly recommended. I felt that it could be nothing but advantageous to support my overall well-being and body's natural processes with herbal medicine.

Jenny was also an iridologist and I was curious what she would reveal from the secrets in my eyes. I loved Jen and her intriguing treatments; it was the first of many visits to her over a 12 month period. If nothing else, the quiet times I had with Jen in her Zen hut gave me an opportunity to share my feelings, and I felt comforted knowing she had my back on this scary journey. My cycle was sort of starting to regulate and Jen reassured me it was quite normal for it to take this long, and also absolutely normal for it to take up to 12 months to conceive after coming off the pill. Regardless of what she or anyone else said, I was definitely feeling the urgency to conceive as soon as possible. In my mind there was no time to waste.

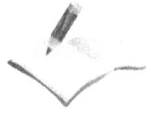

17/08/11 CYCLE DAY 12

I have been experiencing a huge sense of overwhelm in the past few weeks which has left me feeling dizzy, tired and stressed. From the outside I probably look 'normal' but I don't feel that way on the inside. Reading back through past entries reveals this is not new for me, which I know isn't. Hopefully as I've gotten older, I recognise the signs earlier and know how to handle myself a little better. Can you believe I'm 30 now?! I saw a herbalist today for the first time and she was excellent. She mentioned a few areas in my body that need supporting – my bowel, ovaries and thyroid. So, I have some bloody awful tasting drops to take now. The great news is that Jenny said she can't see anything stopping me from falling pregnant and that I should be pregnant within a few months of treatment, providing I don't conceive this month. She asked me to promise her that so the drops have time to work and produce the right environment for our baby. Adam and I are so looking forward to being parents. I went off the pill in October last year after our wedding, and nothing has happened as yet. I had started to feel worried and negative about that, but seeing Jenny today has made me feel better and given me hope that it will happen. Tomorrow is the first day of month two of ovulation tests, so I'll see how that goes as well.

18/08/11 CYCLE DAY 13

Day 1 of ovulation tests today and nothing as yet. It did cross my mind today that the company that manufactures the kits might make them all read negative so we keep on buying them and making them money. Surely not? The herbal potion I got from the herbalist tastes absolutely dreadful, but it has to be good for me. After months of trying to conceive it's going to be interesting/weird trying not to conceive this month. I spoke to Adam tonight about him going to see the herbalist and he was halfway receptive, which was a surprise. Well it is bedtime now and I need a rest. Love B xo

19/08/11 CYCLE DAY 14

No purple strip on the little stick today, though I did leave it sitting on the floor for 20 minutes and forgot to check it. Woops. I can't bring myself to try not to fall pregnant for the herbalist lady. I figure that we've been trying for 10 months for something to happen, and it hasn't, so surely nothing will happen this month. Feeling better about life today and going to bed at 10:45pm on a Friday night. I must be getting old. B xo

20/08/11 CYCLE DAY 15 12:51am

Have just picked Adam up from a bucks party and now hitting the hay. He's in surprisingly good shape – almost sober it seems, with a few bruises from paint ball. I've had a busy day working on a market research final report, doing housework and jobs and packing. Nothing on the ovulation stick... do I really not ovulate or is the test wrong? B xo

22/08/11 CYCLE DAY 17 10:38pm

Day 5 of the ovulation tests and nothing... No wonder this does my head in! A colleague told me today that she is six weeks pregnant after she and her husband have been trying for 18 months. I'm so excited for her and this gives me hope. I don't really like the word 'trying' – who would have thought you'd have to 'try' to do one of the most natural things in the world. It's so bizarre. I've had a massive day of work today – 11.5hrs – but it was successful – I completed one bull sale campaign and submitted a market research report (67 pages!) that Maria and I have been working on together.

04/09/11 CYCLE DAY 30 10:34pm

Day 30 and I feel like I could be pregnant. I've had a funny discharge I don't usually get and I feel so bloated. However, I've been in this position before and sometimes pre-menstrual symptoms are so similar to pregnancy symptoms. And... these days I don't really know my body or what a 'normal' cycle is. I've been feeling like I'm going to get my period for the past few days and nothing yet. Anyway, all I can do is wait and see.

08/09/11 CYCLE DAY 2 10:46pm

Nature dealt her cruel blow yesterday and I got my period. Sigh. Sometimes I feel like it will never happen to us, though I'll pick myself up again and be positive that it will happen this month.

. . .

Amongst the trying a lot there were some major changes brewing behind the scenes for Adam and I. In May 2011, an exciting career opportunity presented itself for Adam: a Farm Manager/On-Farm Agronomist position with a corporate agricultural company in central/southern NSW. Although Adam had begun to insinuate that he may like a change soon, he wasn't actively seeking a new job. I feel like the job came looking for him because as soon as I came across the advertisement in *The Land* newspaper it felt like a good fit for us.

We had been farming some land near Adam's parents at Grong Grong with Adam's older brother Nathan for nearly two years. If we moved for this new position, we would be living a lot closer to Grong Grong and be able to share more in the farm work. The opportunity for Adam to progress in his career, for us to be more involved in the farming, and closer to one side of our family was very appealing.

Conversely, there were some fairly substantial stumbling blocks from my perspective: my business, moving further from my family and leaving Gunnedah where we enjoyed living and had established our life together. We had some big decisions to make. It was a very stressful time, mostly for me, as I had been putting my heart and soul into growing my business there. Only the month before I had taken on Sunburnt Country Consulting's first full time employee – Maria – in addition to a team of contractors. She wasn't just any old employee either, she was a special friend who chose to come and work with me (and took a pay cut) when she moved back to the bush. She had other options, but we knew that together we would make a good team and do really great work. I had recently invested a substantial amount of money and resources into getting our 'real' office set up. It was a big deal to introduce a full-time wage into the mix and I knew we were going to need some solid client contracts and projects quick smart to cover the increase in overheads. They were in the pipeline but there was a period of time skating on thin ice when the pressure was intense to generate more income on a consistent basis. I still feel sick to the stomach thinking about that time. The turmoil within me was gut-wrenching. How could we move and abandon all I had built when I had just crossed the threshold and moved into the next growth phase of business? How could I let my team down? And was it what I really wanted? Of course, I was planning (hoping) that there would soon be a pregnancy and baby in the picture so that weighed heavily on my mind.

Adam and I thoroughly considered every option for the future. Could Sunburnt Country continue as it was in Gunnedah with me working remotely? Should I engage a manager and step back to concentrate more on client work? Should I give it all away and get a job if we moved? Or should I simply downsize? There was so much to evaluate.

When it came to the crunch there were a few things that were the clinchers. This was my thinking at the time:

a) If I was going to have a baby and be a stay-at-home Mum working part-time, then Adam was the main breadwinner and the employment package he was presented with was hard to turn down. We also had our farming enterprise to consider, which in the previous year had been nicely profitable. For the security of our future family, Adam's job had to come first. He was going to be bringing home the bacon, so to speak.

b) To help our chance of conceiving, I had to reduce my stress. After focusing on my business so intently for so long what I wanted more than anything was to have a baby. I thought it was time to take it a little easier. On top of that, I knew there were some hard yards to do to get Sunburnt Country over the growth hump. That wasn't exactly conducive to less stress.

c) I didn't think it would work (for me, with my personality) long term being remote from my team and I didn't want an 'outsider' managing Sunburnt Country in my place. It had become evident that being a good manager and being good at your craft are two very different things and none of the team wanted, or were skilled to take on the management of the business. Plus, it wasn't financially viable to pay a manager as well as me.

In the end Adam and I made the tough decision that he would take the job and we'd relocate. I decided to trim Sunburnt Country back to a few core clients that I could account manage myself, and there were some projects that I could continue to collaborate on with a few of the Sunburnt team members. Sharing this news with the girls was challenging and emotional. The 'sorry, I have to let you go' conversation with Maria was one of the hardest things I have ever done.

It was a strained time packing up the office, letting our clients know Sunburnt Country's new direction, and the girls finishing up one by one. I had *just* by the skin of my teeth got to where I wanted to be in my business and begun a new chapter. I didn't get the chance to see it evolve and go to the next level. I grieved over the hours of hard work and low income as a new business that I didn't get to capitalise on. It wasn't completely the end, but it was the end of an era. I felt sadness and resentment, but also some relief that maybe this was what I needed to do to fall pregnant. Maybe this was the key! Sunburnt Country was downsizing but this plan lent itself to building the shared dream Adam and I had of living on the land with an agricultural business.

On the eleventh of October 2011, with the help of Adam's parents, we moved ourselves 580km south to a house in the middle of an 8000 acre wheat paddock at Back Creek in central NSW. So much space. And a lovely brick home to make our own. A new adventure. As we drove away from Gunnedah, I put on a brave face and convinced myself of all the positives. I'd get used to it.

In my head I was doing the right thing for our future family. I didn't let myself listen to my heart – it was saying we were driving in the wrong direction.

CHAPTER 3

Trying and succeeding

Trying took a backseat during the month of October 2011 as we packed up and moved all our possessions and two dogs Jo (Border Collie) and Bella (black Kelpie X) to our house in the middle of the wheat paddock at Back Creek. I was still taking the dreadful tasting drops from my herbalist, but there was no temperature plotting, ovulation tests or timing of anything that month while we were consumed with the move. In fact, any sort of 'lovin' was scarce during the month of October. It was a surprisingly welcome break to take our focused attention off it.

As lovely as it was, the house we moved into had been used as a farm worker's quarters for a while so needed to be thoroughly cleaned before we (read I) could begin to unpack. And it was a big house. Adam started his new job as soon as we arrived, so life began at full throttle there and that's how it continued. I had taken the month off work to set about the task ahead – cleaning, unpacking, exploring the property with my dogs and setting up the office which was now a shared space with Adam. There's a lot of logistical stuff to organise when you move, like updating addresses and setting up telecommunications (particularly frustrating when living in the bush!), so there was no shortage of things to do.

We lived approximately 25 minutes from the small town of West Wyalong which was to become our base for everyday supplies like groceries, mail and pharmacy items. I knew one person there – a friend from college, so it was exciting to see her again and meet her husband, who, coincidentally, went to college with Adam. In time I wanted to become involved in the West Wyalong community.

By contrast, the town of Temora became Adam's main community as that's where his office was and where he played rugby. It was a 45-minute drive on back roads from our place to Temora. It was about an hour to the larger town of Young, one and a half hours to our farm near Grong Grong, and two hours to the major regional centre of Wagga Wagga.

This was the beginning of our five year plan:

1. To enjoy making this our new home
2. For Adam to really sink his teeth into his new job, progress in his career and earn good money
3. For me to continue working in my business until having a baby
4. For us to keep building our farming enterprise in conjunction with Adam's family (and earn more good money)

Simple. The perfect plan.

I felt quite optimistic about the plan and committed to it on a surface level. It was a mammoth transition, but I'm good at doing busy so I burrowed in to my to-do list to see me through it.

There was an ever-present question: how long will it be before I am pregnant? Moving is classified as one of life's most stressful events, so I had zero expectation of pregnancy news any time around our relocation. I did hope, however, that the change in circumstances regarding my business would mean less stress and improved chances. Only time would tell.

Three months prior I had seen my gynaecologist in Queensland for ongoing consultation and we discussed Adam and I trying for a baby. She thought we needed to give it more time, but given my history of endometriosis, and while she and I were in the same room (for the last time, it turns out), we discussed options to assist conceiving – if I wished to pursue them. The first of them was some cycle tracking and taking Clomid® to stimulate ovulation. At the time I decided to delay it but as soon as we moved, I was ready to start Clomid. I always felt better with a plan in place... perhaps because it gave me a (false) sense of being in control of the situation.

The plan was to start taking one Clomid tablet a day on the morning of Day 2 of my cycle, through Day 6, followed by a follicle tracking scan on Day 10. I found out where I could have a follicle tracking scan in Wagga Wagga and got everything organised to get underway on my next cycle. Yes! We were back on track.

With Clomid there's a slight increased risk of producing twins due to possibly releasing more than one egg at ovulation and subsequent fertilisation of more than one egg. It wasn't of concern to us and certainly not something we dwelled on as the statistics were well in favour of a singleton pregnancy. We didn't ever focus too much on the topic of twins; I didn't have strong feelings about it either way. A set of fraternal twins in Adam's extended family were the only twins in either of our families. We were aiming for one baby and if we got two, well that would be a bonus.

So, the plan was in place and now all I had to do was wait until my period arrived. I hadn't been as focused on it this month as I usually was, but I couldn't *not* wonder whether this would be *the* month we'd have our good news. It's impossible not to do that when you're trying. You cannot escape from the time bomb counting down to D-day (or more aptly, P-day?) in your brain.

As usual, as the due date neared, I began to analyse my pre-menstrual symptoms – of which I used to get plenty, including cramps, lower backache, mood swings and spotting. It's a special kind of mental anguish, taunting you with every pre-menstrual symptom that could also possibly be a pregnancy symptom. It's like a see saw has set up residence, with Mrs. Rational sitting on one end and Mrs. Optimistic on the other. Sometimes the see saw was equally weighted and in fluid motion. At other times, particularly when hormones were playing their part late in the month, it went wildly up and down. The internal dialogue on the see saw went a bit like this:

That cramp feels a little different this month, maybe I'm pregnant!
Don't jump the gun.

But it feels like it's a bit more in my ovaries and I didn't have this cramp on this day last month.
Don't get your hopes up. We've been here before remember.

Oh my God what about if I am pregnant!
Just see what happens, we'll cross that bridge when we get to it.

Why can't I just be pregnant like everyone else!?
It will happen when the time is right.

Hmmm how long will I leave it before I do a pregnancy test this month…
Be patient!

Should I mention it to Adam?
No.

Then I would proceed to Google 'early pregnancy symptoms' for the 800th time.

It was typical for my periods to be irregular and my cycle to stretch beyond 32 days, so I tried not to let my thoughts run away once I got past that point. The days did seem to drag by ever so slowly though.

I had a home pregnancy test in the bathroom cupboard (of course I did) and I made the very well-considered decision to do a test on day 35 if my period still hadn't arrived. The see saw conversation was amplifying, but I did my best to quiet Mrs. R. and Mrs. O. This wasn't my first rodeo – I had had months of wondering, waiting and hoping, only to be crushed with disappointment.

On day 34, I noticed twinges in my ovaries and a little bit of pain in my lower back and abdomen several times during the day.

I willed the daylight to come each time I woke with anticipation during the night between day 34 and day 35. I was on standby to do the pregnancy test first thing in the morning (the time of day most likely to show pregnancy hormone in your urine). I expected to see blood on the paper every time I went to the toilet in the week leading up to this, but there was still nothing, so maybe… just maybe…

It was a Saturday morning. I woke early while Adam slept, snuck quietly into our ensuite and closed the door so he wouldn't hear me open the box and unwrap the stick from its plastic packaging. I was hiding it from him because if it was negative, I didn't want to hear his words again, along the lines of – "why do you get your hopes up, why don't you just wait a bit longer?" Also, if it was negative, I'd do another test the following morning and not want him to know about that either. He thought I was putting myself through unnecessary anguish, and wasting money. If only he knew. I deliberated over buying pregnancy tests in bulk but could never bring myself to do it because it seemed like I was then inviting infinite pregnancy testing into my life.

With heart pounding, I peed in a plastic cup and carefully followed the instructions as I always did, dipping the plastic test stick into the urine for the precise amount of time (timed on my phone). There was no way I was going to bugger up and get the pregnancy test procedure wrong. I preferred to pee in the cup and dip the stick in rather than urinating directly onto the stick in the toilet – just in case I didn't aim well enough!

We had been trying to fall pregnant for 11 months at this point and I had done plenty of home pregnancy tests. It is a cruel exercise. I don't know if words can do justice to the conflicting emotions coursing through your body – the hope, the anxiety, trying to stay detached from the outcome, but desperately, *desperately* wanting to see those two pink lines. I vacillated between convincing myself it would be negative and already imagining my swollen belly. This was no exception.

I would always debate whether to stay and watch the results window or walk away and come back to it. Most of the time I couldn't tear my eyes away – I would stare at it with adrenalin surging, heart racing, almost physically ill, one eye on my phone timer as I watched the control line appear like magic (great, the test is working) and the liquid heading for the test result window. I would tell myself "No matter what the test result is, I'll be Okay." If it was negative after the required three minutes, I'd say to myself, "It could still be coming" so I'd leave and distract myself up to the maximum 10 minute mark. I was kidding myself. I would come back to it, gather myself, and throw it in the bin along with my hopes for that month. I liked to push it well down in the bin so Adam didn't see it – to protect both of us.

Not this morning. This time it was a digital test and within one minute it flashed up PREGNANT 1 - 2 weeks. Oh my God. Oh my God. OH MY GOD. Eyes wide, my hand over my mouth, a moment in time to savour. With utter elation and disbelief, I ran, shrieking, into the bedroom to show Adam the test. Our smiles and embrace were supercharged. Right there in that instant, the possibilities open up and forever you, and your entire future, are transformed. Adam was quick to chime in with the "let's not get carried away, it's early days" comments, which I took on board, but if we couldn't be a little excited now than when could we be?

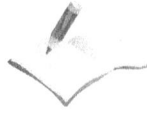

13/11/11 12:10am CYCLE DAY 35

This morning my home pregnancy test said:

PREGNANT

1-2 weeks

I couldn't believe it and hardly dare to believe it. On Monday I'll book in with a doctor for a blood test to confirm. Neither Ad nor I want to get our hopes up too high, but it's hard not to when you get a positive test result! I was waiting for my period to start my first course of Clomid, followed by a follicle scan on Day 10. Seems like nature may have found its own way. How so cliché that friends said I would fall pregnant when we moved... and wallah! I do feel as though I am pregnant – I have funny feelings in my ovaries and tummy. Here's hoping all is okay. It would fill the void I am feeling in my life. Might read my book for a little while now and wait for Ad to get home. I am missing him so much – he's working long and odd hours at the moment.

. . .

Two pink lines. Or in this case the word PREGNANT. It astounded me then, and still does, that in the space of one moment you go from being not pregnant to pregnant. From being just you to being two of you. From being a woman to being a mother. From pregnancy being a hypothetical, to it being a reality. You go from clinging to hope that you'll create a baby, to clinging to hope that you'll keep it. And just like that you're thrust into the next chapter of your life and you are fantasising over due dates, which doctor you'll use, where you'll deliver and is it a boy or girl. It is *the* most incredible, scary, wonderful feeling. If the feeling was a manmade drug, addiction would be rife.

Finally, our wait was over and what's funny is that all of a sudden, the trying felt distant and irrelevant... we were going to be parents.

I found a pregnancy due date calculator online, entered my cycle length and date of the first day of my last period, and it revealed the due date for our baby: 20 July 2012. A winter baby!

Adam went to work that day and I floated around on cloud nine wondering what to do with myself. I wasn't meant to tell anybody yet, so I revelled in the joy alone and spent the morning researching early pregnancy. I was determined that being pregnant wasn't going to stop me from doing things, so I didn't see the need to rest that weekend. Instead, that afternoon I mowed the grass with the push mower in the late spring heat, practically gliding over the lawn in bliss. I repeated in my head, "we are having a baby; we are having a baby." That night I did NOT have wine and I was giddy at the joy in that simple turn of events.

It was beyond ironic to me that we had conceived during such a stressful time. It was illogical and frustrating. I hated that it satisfied the "it will happen when you least expect it" notion that so many people had willingly shared with us. Was that how it really worked – you can try so hard and get nowhere and when you don't try it happens? What are you meant to do – try, or not try? I couldn't equate it, but right now it did not matter and I could shake my head and wonder, 'how the bloody hell did that just happen?'

I called the Temora Medical Centre as soon as it opened Monday morning and made an appointment for later that day to obtain a blood test referral. I had the belief that it wasn't truly real until a blood test confirmed it, so that's what I was hanging out for. I didn't want to have another day of not being sure. At this point I had no symptoms other than the sort of abdominal and lower back cramping I usually experienced with my period.

I saw a lovely female GP who established with a urine test that yes, it did appear I was expecting (big grin from me, of course). She quickly launched into all the routine pregnancy information about folic acid, rest, what I should and shouldn't eat, antenatal care, what to expect when pregnant, etc. It felt surreal. I was vaguely taking it in while at the same time high-fiving myself, 'WOOHOO I AM IN THE BABY CLUB!' She also cautioned that it was early days and talked about the risk of miscarriage. Although I was very aware of the possibility of miscarriage, the swing in the conversation from nurturing a life to preparing for death threw me off balance for a moment or two. I needed to hear it, but I didn't want to. I was ready for this and it was meant to be, for goodness sake!

On leaving her office and heading to the pathology centre down the road, I was a bundle of emotions. I was desperate to get the result and confirm this was really happening, and I could tell my family!

I rang for the result on Tuesday morning and received the ultimate news that based on my human chorionic gonadotropin (hCG) level I was about five weeks pregnant. Wow, Wow, WOW! Nothing could wipe the smile off my face that day. When Adam got home that afternoon, we rang the members of my immediate family to share our news, and agreed that we'd wait to tell his family in person. It was harvest time so we'd see them at the farm soon enough.

I was divinely happy in those first days of knowing I was pregnant, but it wasn't long before I was desiring the 12 week mark. I wished I looked and felt pregnant and could tell people. Where was the morning sickness and the belly!? I wanted all of it. While you have no choice but to take it day-by-day when you're pregnant, there is an unmistakeable urge to want to fast-track it past those risky early weeks. I reminded myself to relish every moment and at the same time was wishing the days away. This was another journey beyond my control that I couldn't project manage the shit out of. I was going to have to learn to live more in the present.

Because of the demands of harvest, Adam was working all day every day for his employer. As the weekend drew near, we realised he'd be unable to help harvest the crops at our farm. I suggested that I could drive down Saturday and drive the chaser bin for the weekend to help out. We only momentarily questioned whether it was the right thing for little old pregnant me to do. Knowing that I would be sitting in the air conditioned comfort of the tractor, we agreed it should be fine. In Adam's absence, I'd head down to lend a hand. I always enjoyed it and it would be a good thing to help a few more days pass towards the 12 week milestone!

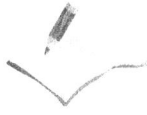

16/11/11

We are having a baby! We are so blessed and can't believe it's happening to us, without any assistance. I got my blood and urine test results back yesterday afternoon and all was good. I have told Mum and Dad, Kylee, Shawn, Terri and Grandma, and we are going to wait to tell Ad's family in person in the next few weeks. Apparently, I am 4-5 weeks pregnant. Feeling tired today and my boobs are starting to hurt! Early to bed for me tonight. Ad is harvesting. He started at 7pm and will work through to 7am. He is so proud and excited. I pray that everything happens as it should now. Love from pregnant Louey.

CHAPTER 4

Trying to understand

On the morning of Saturday the nineteenth of November 2011, I rose early and drove to Grong Grong to assist with harvest on our farm and Adam's parents' farm. I'd not done any hands-on farm work down there without Adam so I was a teeny bit anxious, for no good reason other than that it was new to go on my own. Now that I was predominantly a pencil pusher in an office, I also worried that my common sense had disappeared and I might do something wrong. When you don't operate machinery very often it can take a while to regain your judgement of speed and distance, and also be switched on to be a proficient operator. Naturally I wanted to do a good job (and not wreck any gear)!

I felt a bit uncomfortable that Adam's family didn't know I was pregnant, but we had decided we'd share the news together and it could wait until I was a little further along – maybe seven or eight weeks. I also didn't want them to think differently of me or stop me from helping out. I wonder if I seemed strange to them that day. I certainly felt it, trying to carry on as per normal while keeping the big secret that threatened to explode out of me.

We got into the day, with me driving the tractor that pulls the chaser bin. Chaser bin is the name of the portable bin the combine harvester (or header as we refer to it) empties its grain into on the run. Late in the afternoon we moved the header and chaser bin to another property on which Adam's Dad and brother were to start contract harvesting. I thought about Adam as the day went on, wondering how he was doing harvesting on one of the properties owned by the company he worked for. He was putting in big hours and I hardly saw him.

I felt a bit tired and 'off' all day, but not enough for me to think too much of it. Maybe that's how you were meant to feel in early pregnancy? I actually felt comforted by it initially. The day was busy, hot and I spent a good deal of time bouncing around in the ute and tractor, so I wasn't surprised that I felt exceptionally worn out when I walked into the house about 6pm. There was a greeting party. As is the norm for harvest time, there were extra hands on deck to help out, and on this day it was an Uncle and cousin of Adam's from Victoria. My two young Bensch nephews were also staying at the house that night.

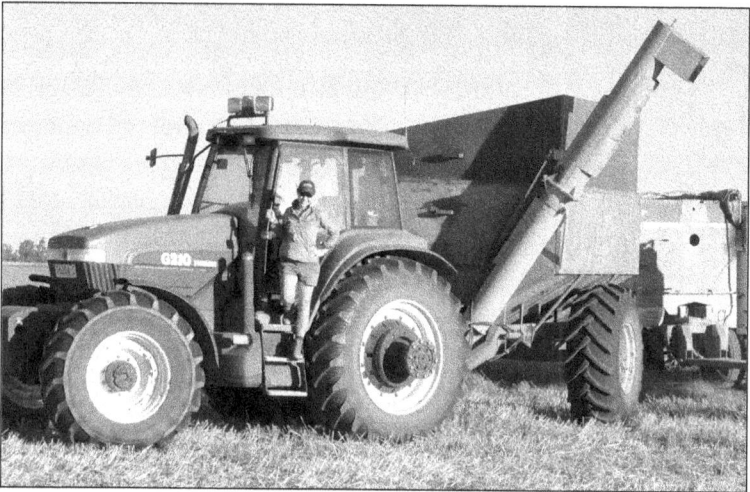

From pencil pusher to chaser bin driver, Grong Grong November 2011.

Soon after getting inside, at about 7pm, I began to notice an achiness in my lower back and abdomen, not dissimilar to mild period pain. I showered, had dinner, chatted to Adam's Mum and tried not to read into it. As the evening wore on, the achiness worsened and by 10pm I was having proper cramps. Shit.

My first reaction: I need Adam. In stealth mode I went to the kitchen to get the cordless landline phone, then dialled his number from the bedroom I was staying in. But there was no mobile phone service where he was, so it went straight to his voicemail again and again and again. Shit! Thankfully it was an hour earlier in Queensland so I decided to ring Mum and then

Kylee (a mother of three). I asked both if the cramping was normal, to which they both replied along the lines of "not really," but I only needed to worry if there was bleeding with it. There wasn't. So, there was nothing to do but wait and see what happened overnight. Despite the pain and my fretfulness, I managed to get to sleep about 11pm… silently fearing the worst.

I woke with a start at 2am in quite a lot of pain and needing to go to the toilet. When I wiped there it was – blood. Crimson red blood. Unmoving, I sat and stared at the toilet paper. The harshest reality there was, staring right back at me. Blood – such an essential part of life but in this moment so dreadfully unwanted.

In my head I was screaming "Noooooooooooooo!" but I couldn't make a sound because there were seven sleeping bodies in the house. Not one of them was my husband and not one of them knew I was pregnant. The devastation rose up inside as I knew what this bleeding likely meant. *However*, I started to cling to the hope that it was just a little bleeding that some pregnant women experience. All of the stories I'd heard about this came rushing in and consoled me momentarily.

I went back to the bedroom and sat on the bed, mind whirring, contemplating what to do next. I lay down and waited a little while. Breathe Benita, just breathe. The pain was strong now. I went to the toilet again and there was more blood. This couldn't be happening to me! I still couldn't reach Adam. I needed someone so I tiptoed around the corner to the door of Adam's parents' bedroom to call out for my mother-in-law, Sandy. It took me back to being a little girl, standing in the doorway of my parents' bedroom to get Mum when I was sick or afraid. I'm pretty sure over all those years I perfected the fine art of speaking loudly enough that she would hear me, but not so loud that I would wake Dad. There was also the trying not to sound too panicky, but willing her to recognise the pleading tone in my voice. It came in handy now because I really didn't want Adam's Dad to wake up… this was not a discussion I wanted to have with him under the circumstances.

"Sandy, can I please talk to you?" Thank the Lord, Sandy woke the second time I asked. With characteristic mother bear instinct, she was instantly up and out of bed and we walked into my room which adjoins theirs.

With as much strength as I could muster, I said "Sorry to wake you Sandy, I'm almost six weeks pregnant and I think I'm losing the baby." In that moment I was extremely grateful for my loving mother-in-law. She gave me a sanitary pad and we chatted for about 10 minutes about miscarriage and what I should do. We decided to ring the GP hotline and I spoke to the nurse about what was going on. They recommended I go to hospital.

After some consideration, Sandy and I decided that's what we'd do. We rang the Narrandera Hospital to advise them I was coming in. They said that if I was miscarrying there wasn't much they could do but keep me comfortable, but I could come in if I wanted to and if it helped me feel better. I had read about ectopic pregnancies and other complications, so I wanted to be sure nothing like that was happening. It was also the middle of the night and sitting in a bedroom on my own going through torture while everyone else slept was not appealing. The thought of being in a house full of men while having a miscarriage was *exceedingly* unappealing. I badly wanted Adam. At least at the hospital I could talk freely and have someone to monitor me. We drove the 15 minutes to Narrandera. In the car it was one of those times when you don't want to talk about the obvious, but the obvious is all you can talk about. Yet there's nothing to be gained by continuing to talk so you mostly sit in silence.

We arrived at the hospital about 3am. I was relieved to get there because on the inside I was crumbling into a million pieces. I had passed more blood and had what I'd describe as severe period pain. In my heart I knew what was happening. I was the only patient in the Emergency Department that night so had two nurses to myself to fuss over me. There really was nothing they could do other than monitor my vitals, give me a bed to lie on and Panadol® to relieve the pain. They told me that a midwife would come to see me early in the morning, which was only a few hours away at that stage. Sandy offered to stay but we decided it was best she head home so she was there when the kids woke. After all, there was nothing she could do, and I wanted some quiet time to myself. It was the closest I'd ever felt to Sandy, to share something so personal and also so womanly.

After being there for a little while I needed to relieve my bladder. I had been unconsciously holding it because I desperately did not want to see what I expected would confront me – more blood. It was the feeling I had every month when my period arrived, but multiplied by 1000. If I didn't actually see it, then maybe it wasn't really happening. But then there's that part of you that needs to see it, to know. As I rose off the toilet seat there was a small gush into the water which was a number of large-ish blood clots and tissue. I looked down. What I saw will stay with me forever. There was no actual visual proof but I knew then that we'd lost our baby – in the toilet at the Narrandera Hospital, on my own. So cold and downright awful. I wanted to curl into a ball and howl. But I didn't. I informed the nurses as they had requested that I describe what I was passing – the colour, how much and what size the clots were. Clinical but necessary.

The rest of the night passed with more bleeding and cramping and a few fits of sleep before the midwife arrived as the sun was coming up. She was like an angel sent from heaven – one of those beautiful women with a motherly vibe that you want to allow yourself be enveloped by. I lapped up her beautiful energy while she sat next to my bed and held my hand. She spoke about all the medical stuff and also about the two miscarriages she'd had – both in the second trimester. We chatted about why… why would this happen? She was the first of many people to reassure me that I was the not the cause of what happened, and not to blame myself. That if I did lose the baby, it was probably because there was something wrong and it wasn't mean to be. BUT. Maybe if I had not been jolting around in the tractor working yesterday? Maybe if I had taken it easy and stayed at home? Maybe I overdid it? Or was it something I had eaten? It was impossible not to question, but there were no answers to be found, and there never would be. Another mystery of the universe – just like conceiving felt like to me.

The midwife encouraged me not to give up hope because some women did experience bleeding and remained pregnant. It's what I yearned to hear, yet equally didn't want to. I didn't want to cling onto false hopes; I didn't want to put myself through that. I wanted to know for certain, but I wouldn't know that for several days yet – either via ultrasound or blood test. More of the waiting game. I was finally able to reach Adam on the phone and after being connected by elation only days prior, we were now connected by loss.

The cramping had subsided somewhat and I was due to be discharged at 9am, so I rang Sandy and asked her to please come and collect me. I left the hospital feeling drained and hollow. Back at Adam's parents' house I promptly packed my things. The last thing I felt like doing was making awkward small talk with all the men and the massive white elephant in the room. I hopped in my car and drove the one and a half hours north. I sobbed as I drove, alternating between primal, uncontrollable body-shaking and gentle, silent tears. And then all that was left was a constant dull ache in my heart and head. Adam took the day off and I was longing for the comfort of his big chest and arms, which embraced me intensely when I arrived home. He was as upset as I was, but it was not expressed through his tears – that's not my Adam's style. We took it easy that day and hugged a lot.

Over the next 24 hours, and then several days, the bleeding would ebb and flow in waves. When it was light, I hung on to a tiny, minute sliver of hope, and then it would be heavy and I'd think, "you're kidding yourself Benita, it's over." The next day, on Monday, I saw the same GP who confirmed my pregnancy and she verified via cervical examination that I had miscarried. The following day my hCG level confirmed the same. There was no need for an ultrasound.

In the days and weeks that followed, cruelly, just like the lead up to a period, I experienced what felt like early pregnancy symptoms – back pain, a metallic taste in my mouth, a little nauseous, bloated. I had to be imagining them. I was trying to imagine them into life. Or could there be some bizarre possible way that the doctor and blood test were wrong? Unfortunately, that wasn't the case.

I was extremely frustrated by the prospect of waiting another six, eight or 12 months or however long before becoming pregnant again. If ever! Every month felt like forever and made me one month older. I now had a whole new bunch of questions to stew on, like:

Will I fall pregnant again?

Will I miscarry again?

Why did I miscarry?

Did I cause it?

It's not just about losing a baby, it's also the loss of hope and faith, and losing a part of you too.

At this time, I realised that trying to conceive was only the first step of the end goal. After that came staying pregnant with a healthy baby, and finally bringing him or her safely into the world. You had to win one stage at a time. Looking ahead seemed insurmountable.

To add insult to injury, I already had a lot of hand-me-down baby items and clothes from Kylee sitting in the room that was to be the nursery. I had to shut the door.

After a few days of feeling deeply sad, I did my best to get going again. The grief and disappointment were unrelenting, but moping for too long is not my way. As always, work was a great distraction, and there was an abundance of that to do. Christmas was also approaching and we were heading up to Queensland to share it with my family. I was looking forward to it immensely. I knew that some Davis family time was just what I needed.

What a start to our time at Back Creek – the big move, Adam starting his job, setting up our new house, harvest at Grong Grong, discovering I was pregnant, and then losing our baby – all in the space of five weeks. At the time I didn't take stock of the enormity of it; I just kept on moving as best I could. But a small piece of me was broken... and always will be.

In the lead up to Christmas we planted a lemon tree just outside our backyard for the baby that was all at once ours, but never ours. It was symbolic for me and gave me a place to go to feel, and to talk to the spirit of our little one whom we had nicknamed Ronnie Bean Bensch. A lemon tree was the perfect choice as I later came to learn that lemons clear away negative energy and have the power to heal.

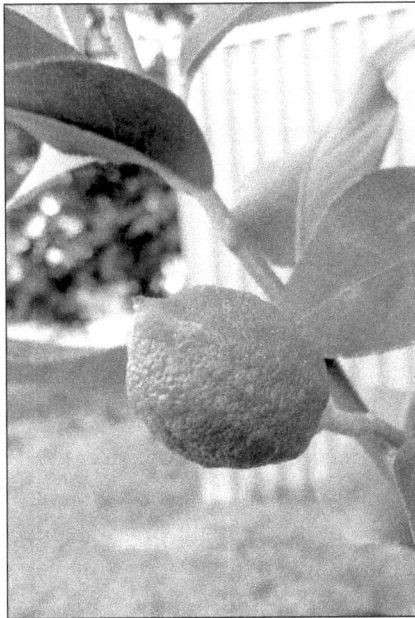

The lemon tree we planted in honour of Ronnie Bean – the baby I carried briefly, but never held.

49

A special note on miscarriage

I believe miscarriage is one of the hardest, most bewildering and misunderstood events that can happen in a person's life.

It happens all the time. One in five women who know they are pregnant will have a miscarriage before 20 weeks. The actual rate of miscarriage is even higher than that due to women having very early miscarriages before knowing they are pregnant. I didn't think I'd be in the one in five, but I was, and I could reel off the names of many women in my life who have also miscarried once, or more. I'm sure you can too. In most cases the cause of miscarriage is unknown – thought to be an abnormality with the chromosomes (genes). Miscarriage is nature's way of dealing with it.

Nature's way of dealing with it. This phrase is comforting as well as harsh. And that's how it is with miscarriage – comforting in that my body (nature) knew what it was doing discarding the embryo, but the 'dealing with it' aspect brings the harshness of loss.

The medical fraternity will say that what we lost was *not* a child, it wasn't even classified as a foetus at that point. It was the 'products of conception.' I accept that when they told me this in hospital it was only to help me feel better about the situation. Academically I know that it was only a bunch of cells and tissue. But was our 'products of conception' not worthy of my tears?

In every broken piece of my heart, I felt we had lost a child. *We* lost a child. We *lost* a child. We lost *a child*. Our child.

For one week I got to experience the pure joy of being pregnant. During that time it was pretty much all I could think about and all I wanted to think about. Like a soft warm blanket, I wanted to wrap myself up in it and feel the beauty of it, over and over again. I wanted to roll around in the bliss, bask in it and hide away with it, all to myself. For so long I had wanted to feel it, and, when I did, it was better than I had imagined.

For one week I imagined his sweet little face, touching his perfect soft skin and breathing in the unmistakeable, addictive baby smell. For one week, I pictured myself up in the night breastfeeding him, holding him, kissing his forehead, pushing him in the pram when we went out as a family of three. I was gleaming with pride and happiness as we walked along. I had begun to plan the nursery and started a mental checklist of what I'd need to prepare before his arrival. I could picture my bulging belly, smiling as I rubbed the spot where he was kicking me. I wanted to go through labour, I wanted to be the tired mother of a newborn, I wanted to experience all of it.

Now there was nothing except a throbbing emptiness, more cramps and a bloody reminder every time I went to the toilet. Oh, and the general sense that I should dismiss how I was feeling because it was just 'the products of conception' and it happens all the time.

The topic of miscarriage is handled poorly in our society. Usually when we encounter a loss on life's journey it's broadcast and people come together to show their support. When someone loses a pet and they post the news on social media, the outpouring of condolences is quite profound. When a friend or family member passes it's publicised, openly discussed, the deceased's life is celebrated and people generally support those who are grieving the most.

Yet when you lose a baby before the people in your life and general public know you're pregnant, you suffer in silence. You play it down or hide it away completely. You're a bit distant for a few months and no one knows why. You deactivate your social media account because you can't bear to see another damn pregnancy announcement (mine stayed deactivated for three years).

I questioned:

Was I being dramatic being this upset?

Was I allowed to feel this way?

Was I qualified to talk to other people about miscarriage because ours happened early on?

It was difficult to decide whether I should or shouldn't share with others what had happened. On one hand, I felt I couldn't speak openly and freely about it because of the judgement, or perceived risk of it. On the other, I felt like I needed to validate where I had been and why I was behaving the way I was. I had a lot of conflicting emotions.

I didn't want to appear ungrateful because, after all, I *did* fall pregnant, and I should be grateful for that shouldn't I?

I didn't want to complain, because someone else always has a worse story than our own, so I should just be grateful, shouldn't I?

I didn't want to mention it because it made others feel uncomfortable.

I didn't want to mention it because I didn't want to deal with others reactions and emotions.

I didn't want to mention it because I didn't trust myself enough to know how I might react to their reaction.

I didn't want to mention it because doing so meant feeling it all again.

I didn't want to mention it because it made me question if there was something wrong with my body.

I didn't want to mention it because it made me wonder if I did something wrong to cause it.

I didn't want to mention it because then people would know it had been X months since the miscarriage, and therefore be speculating that we were trying again.

Not only was I telling myself things like, "you were only five and a half weeks, some people lose their babies at full term, you should be grateful that's not you," some people that I did confide in made comments like:

"You just need to relax and it will happen again."

"Well at least you know you can get pregnant."

"It wasn't meant to be."

"At least it was early."

Yes, there was some truth in these statements and I know that people never mean harm in what they say in these circumstances. However, a little more thought and compassion from people wouldn't go astray. All that's needed is "I'm sorry for your loss." That's really it.

Something doesn't sit right with me about the social norm of waiting until 12 weeks gestation to share the news that you are pregnant. We're conditioned to believe this and most people go along without question – including me in the beginning. It sets us up to keep miscarriage hidden and for its wounded to endure their struggle alone. Can't we be as open about miscarriage as we are about celebrating pregnancy?

Can't we rejoice in the joy of conception and respectfully share the pain of loss, like we do with other losses in our life? I couldn't fully comprehend why I was being encouraged not to tell anyone about our pregnancy news before 12 weeks. Shouldn't they know, because if I did lose the baby wouldn't I need support from them? Wouldn't it be a good thing for people to know and be able to provide comfort?

I completely respect people's right to choose in all situations. I am merely exploring this issue so that miscarriage might be treated with more respect and openness.

My conditioning told me to get over it and move on.

I've moved on, but I'll never be over it nor do I need to be.

CHAPTER 5

Trying when your best isn't good enough

2011 had been a HUGE year, so when the New Year rolled around it felt like a clean slate – an opportunity to start afresh. The break over Christmas reminded me there was lots to be grateful for, and I wanted to give it my best shot to embrace our new life down south.

I had some great work projects lined up for the year and Adam was committing himself to his job, and his rugby. On top of that, we spent as much time as we could on our farm. I joined the Events West Wyalong committee as a volunteer to be involved in the community and meet more people. I also looked into playing women's soccer (which I love) in Temora, but decided it wasn't worth registering since I could be pregnant soon, and it would mean travelling distances both days on a weekend – for Adam's rugby Saturday and my soccer on Sunday.

After a month off from trying after losing Ronnie Bean, TTC was back on the agenda in January. I was excited at the prospect of a baby in 2012 and I'd been giving Google a work out with questions like 'chance of falling pregnant after miscarriage.' I pondered whether there was some factor at play which would enhance my fertility after miscarriage because someone had suggested that once (no truth to it by the way). It was a relief to know I could actually get pregnant, though I still wasn't sure how the timing had worked out, and without any planning. Fancy that. Just like other people.

I was fearful that we'd be in for many months of trying again. But surely things would fall into place more quickly now that I'd been pregnant, albeit briefly? Surely. I was cautiously optimistic about what would happen next. It was back to the painfully familiar contradictory headspace where you are hopeful, but you try not to get your hopes up too much. Everything felt slightly different though, after what we'd experienced. The goal was ultimately the same, but I wasn't quite the same person.

We resumed 'activities' around the middle of my cycle when I *thought* I was ovulating. I was recording mucus observations (still gross, stressful and subjective) in my diary.

I decided it was time to take matters into my own hands and get moving on a plan again. None of this sitting and waiting for me. As much as I loved my gynaecologist in Queensland, she was too far away to continue seeing on a regular basis and I wanted to establish a relationship with a doctor nearer to us. I researched gynaecologists in Wagga Wagga and made an appointment to see a female doctor there as soon as possible.

When the day came for my consultation, I explained our story, including that I had endometriosis and was turning 31 that year and didn't want to waste any time. I was hyper aware of the line in the sand at 35 after which the risk of EVERYTHING increases and odds of conception decline. I didn't want to fall into that category if we could help it. I knew that it was more common and 'normal' to have children later, however, when I reflected on the previous generation of women in my life who started having children in their early twenties, 35 seemed so old.

The new gynaecologist and I covered my options and one of them was to do nothing and give things more time. We talked about tracking my cycle and getting a better handle on when I ovulated. We discussed Clomid with its possible side effects, the increased risk of having twins, higher chance of ectopic pregnancy and what the process would involve if we went ahead with it. I had already made this decision months prior, before getting pregnant, so there wasn't much to consider the second time around. The plan was to try Clomid in my next cycle, with a follicle tracking ultrasound scan, and ovulation tests (those bloody things again) to monitor my hormone levels approaching ovulation.

Each Clomid tablet contains clomiphene citrate and is taken daily for five days. Clomid causes the anterior pituitary gland in the brain to release hormones which stimulate ovulation. Like all medications with possible side effects, Clomid has its own list. I really did not enjoy the ones I experienced which were: hot flashes, moodiness, tiredness, anxiety and nervousness. I kept wondering if I was being a hypochondriac and dreaming the symptoms up, but the hot flashes felt pretty real. A massive high five to hot-flashing menopausal women everywhere!

On Day 12 I had a follicle tracking scan which revealed a lovely dominant 21mm follicle on one ovary and other smaller follicles on both ovaries. Yay! Follicles are fluid-filled sacs which contain immature eggs. Normally all of the follicles stop growing except the dominant one which releases a mature egg at ovulation. This was my first, but certainly not my last, glimpse into the phenomenon of watching follicles grow. The gynaecologist was happy with the scan result.

I started ovulation tests on Day 13 and for the next six days they were negative. There might have been a positive on Day 14 as the line was darker, but still not as dark as the control line, so I didn't know what to make of it (face palm). I'm not sure if the emotions I recorded on Days 16 and 17 which included 'crazy mood swings' and 'feeling stressed and angry' were due to the Clomid or the darn ovulation tests. Adam and I were doing 'the deed' regardless of the negative test results, and hoping for the best. From Day 19 through to Day 32 there weren't many days that I didn't record observations like: twinges in my ovaries, lower back pain, pangs in my abdomen, pimples and unusual discharge (which I now know was a result of my endometriosis). I was finely tuned into every little way my body was behaving, to the point of fixation.

During the Clomid cycle, I began to see an acupuncturist to assist with my fertility. I'd had excellent results with acupuncture on my left knee (which apparently is afflicted with rheumatoid arthritis) so I was a big fan. I was increasingly interested in natural therapies to complement western medicine. A friend of mine recommended this particular acupuncturist in Wagga Wagga who she swears helped her conceive, so I decided it was a good starting point.

Her name was Nicole and I was instantly captivated by her aura. She emanated serenity and while I was in her rooms and presence, I trusted that everything was going to be okay. She put me at ease that all was on track and the fact that I had fallen pregnant 10 months into trying was great. Her hands were always warm. As she floated around the bed inserting the acupuncture needles, she'd momentarily place a heavenly hand on my leg, arm or head. During my treatments I felt a calmness in mind and body that I rarely found elsewhere. Except for my first treatment that is. As a result of the Clomid I was so hyped and anxious I found it extremely hard to lie still – which is a problem when you have needles stuck in very specific parts of your body. It was as if I were on speed. I got through it and hoped by some magic that the powers of Clomid and acupuncture would collide to create a super baby.

Unfortunately, there was no super baby and no need for a pregnancy test that month as my period arrived on Day 33. Bugger. Sigh. Stupid Clomid. I decided I was never taking it again.

There was always an upside to the arrival of my period: it heralded Day 1 of a new month. New month = new hope, and at least a few days to take my mind off ovulation and the two week wait coming up. On the first and second day of my period I would work through the process of dealing with the reality that last month wasn't *the* month. And it really was a process – starting with disappointment, then anger, apathy, sadness and ending with a readjustment of my mindset to try again for another month. By the end of Day 2, I'd normally be somewhat back on the wagon and hopeful this could be *the* month.

I continued to see Nicole the acupuncturist and decided I'd commit to acupuncture and her recommended Chinese herbs before pursuing other methods. Over the ensuing four week period I drove the two hours to Wagga Wagga for treatment once a week. It was an effort but I thrived on the proactivity of it, and the calmness the treatments provided me. The cycle day that I was on would influence how Nicole carried out the treatment and where she placed the needles. I felt like she had a special power and I would literally feel the energy radiating through my body from certain needle sites. I imagined the energy from the needles healing and jump-starting parts of my reproductive tract. Well, that's what I was hoping for. I stuck with the intensive period of acupuncture and then saw her as often as I could for many months after that, while continuing with the Chinese herbs at home.

I also started to visit Will the chiropractor who travelled to West Wyalong from his practice in Griffith. Regular chiropractic adjustments had generally been a part of my well-being routine, so it was important to me to continue that in our new town. My initial consultation with Will turned out to be rather intensive and insightful. He took a holistic approach and was interested in what seemed like everything about me except cracking my back, which was the style of chiropractor I was accustomed to. Will is an interesting guy and I am grateful to him for introducing me to new thinking on topics like neurology and mindfulness literature. He facilitated me starting to view my health more holistically, particularly the interaction between mind and body. It was confronting when he suggested that my tendency to want to control situations and the way I handle stress may be linked to my endometriosis and... the miscarriage.

We discussed my history and he asked if there were any particularly stressful events in the past that could have been a trigger for the endometriosis. I thought hard for a moment. There was something. You see, with the glowing list of senior high school achievements that I recounted in Chapter 1, what I neglected to mention was the nervous breakdown that came along with it. The pressure I put on myself to perform academically, in sport, in my numerous leadership and extracurricular roles, at home on the farm, and in my relationships, led to my breaking point. I couldn't complete my year 12 term three biology exam – I walked out, drove home and went to bed for a few days to begin understanding and climbing out of the 'black hole,' as I call it. That was the first of those episodes in my life, and it was a super-sized wake up call. It was the beginning of a lifelong learning journey in self-awareness and self-care. The possibility that the effect of this was linked to conceiving was a sobering thought. I took on what Will said as constructive feedback.

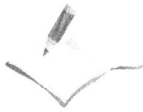

31/03/12 11:18pm

Ad is at Grong Grong tonight for the weekend – cultivating, burning stubble, getting firebreaks ready, picking up logs, all in preparation for planting, which starts in just a few short weeks. Ad has been so busy with his work and the farm; I do hope that he will look after himself in the meantime. I do my best to encourage that, and look after him. Life is also very full for me – my business is going well, mostly with two major clients at the moment. I am preparing full steam ahead for Beef Australia 2012 and the NCHA Futurity, Tamworth. Last week I was in

Tamworth for meetings Thurs/Fri and then in Brisbane Sat-Mon for the Tim McGraw/Faith Hill concert, a meeting and to see my friend and her new baby. Then on Monday night/Tuesday, I visited friends at the Gold Coast with their two little boys. It was wonderful to see Mum & Dad, Kylee & Anthony and Terri for the concert last weekend; I loved it. Overall though, I think I overdid it a bit with the exertion of the whole trip. When I arrived home Tuesday night, I was exhausted. Didn't help that I got my period on Sunday night, accompanied by terrible period pain. I had sore boobs for a week before my period came so I was quietly hopeful I was pregnant. Not to be unfortunately, and it hit me like a ton of bricks... exacerbated by being so tired, and around people all weekend with children. I am now doing my best to let go of any parameters around having a baby. I have been putting so much pressure on myself, and us, since our miscarriage. Now I'm hanging on to the hope, but I'm putting my faith in God that it will happen sometime, somewhere, when it's meant to be. Hard to accept but I have to let go a little or it's going to ruin me, and our marriage. Starting to get sleepy now. Night! B xo

23/04/12 10:52pm

It's bedtime here. Well, for me anyway. Ad is still out there in the darkness, working. I think tonight he is spreading urea. We stayed in Temora Friday night after Ad's rugby game and then went our separate ways Saturday morning – me to Wagga for our nephew's 9th birthday party, and Ad to Grong Grong to the farm. So, this is my 3rd night home alone and probably the first of many. I'm happy in my own company, but only for so long, particularly when I work at home on my own all day. I definitely think too much when I'm on my own, which is what does drive me crazy in the end. Sowing got underway both here and at Grong Grong last Wednesday. There were a few millimetres of rain there last Thursday, which was wonderful, but we do need a little more rain. I'm tired tonight, and have dreadful pre-menstrual tension (PMT) Man I hate it – the bloating and mood swings. The past few days I've been SO emotional – crying over anything! Ads on TV, emails, songs, things I read and think about – pathetic! Hormones really are powerful. My period is due on Thursday and I'm convinced it's coming, again. This lead up is really hard every month but what choice do I have but to get on with it? I hope Ad is safe and warm outside while I'm lying here tucked in bed in my warm PJs. Goodnight. BB xo

As the months rolled on busy with Sunburnt Country work (at home and away) AND acupuncture AND hoping I was ovulating AND hardly seeing Adam AND tracking my cycles down to every possible ovulation and pregnancy/PMT symptom AND recording when we had intercourse AND becoming involved in our new communities AND socialising AND working down at our farm, my frustration slowly began to niggle again.

Was it my endometriosis that was inhibiting us from conceiving? Was it building up again? More than likely it wasn't helping matters! Or was something else going on? Why was this not happening?

Dealing with frustration and lack of control is one of the toughest aspects of trying and getting nowhere. You internalise it and it slowly eats away at you. We are raised under the guise of the old saying "all you can do is your best." I was used to doing my best and achieving whatever I set out to do. Well, when it comes to TTC even your best sometimes isn't good enough. And it sucks. Big time.

I didn't really fit in anymore. I had had my fill of partying and getting drunk on weekends at the pub, races or rugby, but I wasn't yet in the Mum-with-a-pram stage. I was in between in the trying club, and it was a lonely and confusing place to hang. It's a club no one wants to be in and membership should be free because it has shitty benefits. Everyone in it is looking over the fence at the baby club, craving to be with those cool cats instead.

I was grateful to still have my business and great clients, but I discovered that 'work until I get pregnant' was not cutting the mustard in terms of an aspirational business vision. I didn't want to secure any long-term projects in case we had a baby. I didn't know what I could or couldn't take on in case we had a baby. I wasn't setting goals in case we had a baby. A baby was the goal. I felt paused, suspended in motion, just waiting for those two pink lines on the pregnancy test to appear so I could press play on life again. It was stifling.

EVERYTHING hinged on becoming pregnant.

I couldn't see any choice but to remain positive, focus on the day-to-day, keep looking after myself and for Adam and I to keep trying. I was so proud of Adam and admired his commitment to everything he did. However, the weight of his workload took its toll – on him and us. I spent an unhealthy amount of time at home on my own. We also never truly became a part of any one community during our time at Back Creek – we were drifters, and did a lot of driving. It was nothing to do a few hundred kilometres in a day most days of the week.

I turned 31.

Tick, tick, tick.

We had booked a trip to the Northern Territory (NT) in July to visit my cousin and her family, and explore some of the NT. We were looking forward to it immensely – to have a break and to reconnect as a couple. Oh, and maybe while we were in holiday mode, we might be relaxed enough to conceive a baby. Wink wink. Surely if all those other people that conceived on their holidays and honeymoons could do it, we could too. I was eager to find out. I wanted to have a great story to share with our son or daughter like, "Little Johnny/Ruby you were conceived in Kakadu, how cool is that?" I had my fingers crossed.

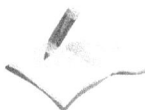

16/07/12

Flying high above the ground somewhere over the middle of the true Australian outback, I ponder life's biggest questions. What is it I really want to achieve? Have I lost sight of my goals? What are my goals? Have I slipped into mediocrity? What am I truly good at? I don't know why flying has always given me perspective. Feeling so far removed from everyday life allows me to think freely and independently of everyday thoughts like 'what have I got to do today'? Today is actually a Monday and I have had to battle the incessant words in my head – 'what have I got to do?' 'where should I be?' 'what deadlines do I have?' 'is there anything I'm forgetting?' It seems these days that I am more at the mercy of my urges to control – to control life, my thoughts, those around me. I often feel worked up without knowing why, how, or that I'm even feeling that way… until I stop. Like today. Until now I haven't been able to shake that feeling of unsettled-ness, if that's a word!? Perhaps because I've spent the last few weeks running and running trying to get 'everything'

*done. But what is everything anyway!? Perhaps I am the reason we
haven't been successful in conceiving and having a child. Perhaps my
body cannot carry a baby because I'm in a heightened state of stress and
don't even know it. My ability to relax certainly has a tarnished record.
Well, I'm looking forward to relaxing on our 2 week holiday in the NT,
split between Darwin, Kakadu and surrounds for 9 days and then Alice
Springs, Uluru and Kings Canyon for 4 days. Speaking of achieving
goals, the in-flight TV just showed the Australian Story documentary
on Black Caviar, the truly amazing mare that has won 21 straight
Group 1 races in Australia, and then won the Royal Ascot Diamond
Jubilee Stakes on 23 June.*

*I think I have a fear of failure and perhaps a little touch of commitment
phobia as well. Why have I felt like I'm stalled for the last while and not
setting goals/making plans? Because I expected we would have a baby
by now and that would be my focus. Having a healthy and happy child
is my goal and would be the greatest gift, and I'm prepared to do whatever is necessary to achieve that goal. Why do I have to make everything
a project? I guess that's just me… We are only 20 minutes from landing
in Darwin now… very excited! xoxo*

. . .

We were disappointed that our fabulous holiday didn't work the baby
magic we were hoping for. So much for "just relax and it will happen!"

Four days into our trip was Ronnie Bean's due date. I ached and cried
for him and what could have been.

In August 2012 we agreed it was time to up the ante. It had been nine
months since my miscarriage and we had been trying (to varying degrees)
for about 19 months in total. I did some research on fertility specialists in
Canberra – our nearest capital city – and we decided on a delightful female
specialist with whom we made an appointment to talk about the next steps.

In summary, the options presented to us were:

a) Be patient and keep trying naturally

b) Give Clomid another go

c) Start ovulation induction (OI) and intrauterine insemination (IUI)

d) Go straight to in vitro fertilisation (IVF).

My perception of IVF was that it was reserved for people at the other end of the spectrum with BAD fertility problems. The last resort. Surely that was not us? It seemed a bit unnatural. And invasive. And scary. And expensive. Although we wanted to help things along, Adam and I decided we didn't want to take that route yet. There was no way I was taking Clomid again, so that left option c. It felt like a nice solution – the next step of assisted conception but not too gung-ho.

Before we could proceed with an OI/IUI cycle, it was compulsory to jump through all the requisite hoops. We had blood tests to verify we were both in tip top health and there were no medical concerns. Check. Adam had to have a sperm test to make sure his swimmers looked and behaved as they should. Check. Adam's health was a very important part of the equation that we hadn't explored. We assumed all was normal enough in that department considering we had conceived naturally once, but it was encouraging to receive Adam's test results which were excellent. Stud sire material. It was a relief to rule out the male factor contributing to our TTC battle. So, it was all on me now… I could deal with that.

The result of my Anti-Mullerian Hormone (AMH) testing weighed heavily on my mind. This test provides an indication of your ovarian reserve. My test result was eight*, which was apparently 'a little on the lower side,' Bam! Okay, I had endometriosis and a low-ish ovarian reserve to contend with. There was no way of knowing about the *quality* of my eggs.

Time for some help. We decided on three consecutive rounds of OI and IUI. We were good to go the following month. I was very enthusiastic about the beginning of a new plan. It meant renewed hope and something to focus on. *Surely*, we would succeed in three rounds.

I later received a letter dated 19th August 2013 from Capital Pathology stating that the company which manufactured the AMH test had notified them some results produced with their test kit were falsely low and have now been shown to be higher on repeat testing. They were concerned my AMH test result might be potentially incorrect and I could have repeat testing if I desired. Yahoo! Maybe my ovarian reserve wasn't so bad after all! I didn't have the repeat test as I figured it didn't really matter anyway – whatever I had in my ovaries to work with was all I was going to get.

CHAPTER 6

Trying with help from our friends

I grew up on a beef cattle farm where inducing ovulation and then artificially inseminating our elite breeding cows was a normal part of life. I was grateful for this upbringing when we started down this path because the process made perfect sense and didn't seem too 'out there' to me. Get the swimmers in the right spot at the right time, let nature take its course and away we go.

I was confident this little bit of assistance would be all we'd need to get us over the line. We could possibly get there on our own again naturally if we were patient enough. But I wasn't.

OI refers to the use of medical therapy to help stimulate the release of an egg when you do not normally ovulate. OI involves taking fertility drugs at the beginning of your cycle – either as tablets or injections – to facilitate follicle stimulating hormone (FSH) which assists the growth and development of the follicles containing eggs. Then, approaching ovulation, blood tests monitor oestrogen and LH levels, and ultrasound scans track follicle development.

My treatment plan consisted of:

- a daily Puregon® (FSH) injection in my stomach starting on Day 2 of my cycle
- a blood test around Day 8
- a blood test and ultrasound scan around Day 10
- potentially another blood test and/or scan around Day 11

- a 'trigger injection' of Ovidrel® at a specific time (as directed) to trigger ovulation,
- the insemination procedure within 48 hours of the trigger
- blood tests seven and 12 days after insemination to monitor oestrogen, progesterone and hCG.

When we travelled to Canberra to collect the drugs for the first cycle, I got to practise injecting an orange to prepare for giving my own injections. Simple, when you're sticking a piece of unflinching fruit. I nervously anticipated the first needle I had to self-administer. When the time came, I had to psyche myself up to actually follow through with it. For ages I sat with my shirt off, using two fingers on my left hand to pinch a fold of alcohol-swabbed skin beneath my belly button, and holding the loaded Puregon pen® in my right hand. Each time I brought it close to my tummy, I pulled it away. Agghh… the anticipation of the sting. There was a lot of cringing and swearing. I tried to convince Adam to do it for me on my virgin attempt, but he refused, which was a good thing because I had to take the plunge at some point. It hurt a little, but wasn't too bad really and I made it a habit to get it done first thing in the morning before overthinking it.

It was nothing compared to what people go through who have acute or chronic illness, and that gave me perspective. This was a new challenge for sure, but I wasn't sick so for that I was exceptionally grateful.

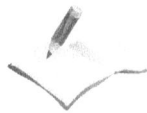

12/09/12 10:39pm [CYCLE 1]

Today I have had my first self-administered injection of Puregon to stimulate ovarian function, which is all part of inducing ovulation. This process will be followed by intra uterine insemination – a procedure we will need to go to Canberra for. We are having 3 cycles of this (OI & IUI) and if unsuccessful we will need to start IVF. I am really hoping that we will conceive in these 3 months. So, since I last wrote, we received the test results and made the decision to proceed with treatment. I am feeling good about this and excited that we are one step closer to an *outcome – our own baby. I achieved a personal milestone on Sunday – I ran 10km in the Canberra Fun Run with my friend Mandy. I have been training for it and my goal was to finish (run the whole way), which I did, in just one hour. It was great fun and it feels good to have achieved a little goal I set myself, while also raising money ($390) for the Royal Flying Doctor Service. This week has been mega busy with work and I have been almost permanently glued to my computer screen. I'm looking forward to getting out and doing something outside on the weekend. We are in need of some rain here to keep the crops going. It's been a harsh cold winter followed by a windy and dry few weeks. People are getting nervous. Goodnight. B xo*

. . .

There were ALOT of blood tests. My farm upbringing also helped in this regard as I had seen plenty of blood. That's not to say I enjoyed blood tests or that I didn't become tired of them. There's no escaping the fact that there's a needle piercing your skin to extract your blood. Sometimes I felt like the life was being drawn out of me. Some blood collection personnel were more skilled than others and I came to know the individuals that I liked in the various collection centres I frequented. It was difficult to find a suitable vein in my arms at times, which could result in several jabs and moving the needle around under my skin to hit the sweet spot. Not particularly fun. Thankfully, I could handle blood tests well without too much apprehension or physical repercussions. I felt for women with an aversion to them; it's hard enough to front up for so many blood tests let alone when you are scared of needles or faint at the sight of blood. I became good at distracting myself while it was happening.

The follicle tracking ultrasound scans were transvaginal so I had to become used to stripping off my bottom half and the sensation of the internal probing. Normally it was uncomfortable, but not painful and lasted 10-30 minutes depending on the technician and what they were finding.

With all the poking and prodding, I began to feel a minor disconnect with my body. It became an instrument of the process to achieve the desired outcome. Whilst I was willing to do whatever it took, it saddened me that creating a baby had become so clinical and a very long way removed from passionate and spontaneous love-making.

Virtually every step in the treatment process was dependent on the result of the previous step, so it was essential to have the blood tests and scans as instructed, and ensure the results were received at the fertility clinic in Canberra by the desired time. This was the bit that frazzled my nerves the most. I had to research where the blood collection centres in our region sent their samples for analysis, and their turnaround times, to have the results back at the clinic in order to make the next decision. There was a bit of trial and error involved in Cycle 1 and 2. Sometimes I'd ring the fertility clinic for my results, and they wouldn't have them, so I'd be urgently chasing the relevant pathology laboratory to send them on. Around this, I was trying to service my Sunburnt Country clients to the best of my ability.

In the end, my system to achieve the optimal least travel/best turn-around time outcome looked like this:

For non-time-critical blood test only: Drive to West Wyalong (25 minutes)
For time-critical blood test only: Drive to Wagga Wagga (2 hours)
For time-critical blood test and scan: Drive to Wagga Wagga (2 hours)
For scan only: Drive to Young (1 hour)

The intensity of the process increased, along with the subsequent effect it had on me, as ovulation drew near. The lack of control I felt with infertility was exacerbated when going through these cycles. Waiting and hoping, waiting and hoping, and life being dictated by what day of the cycle it was. We couldn't make any plans as it got closer to the big O day (ovulation, not orgasm… unfortunately!) so that we were available whenever we needed to travel to Canberra.

It was my first real taste of the challenges associated with undergoing fertility treatment in a rural location. These included: getting drugs delivered to me before I needed them while keeping them chilled, getting blood test results in time so that decisions could be made and the timing precise, driving significant distances multiple times in a cycle and dealing with it all largely on my own. If we had lived in or near Canberra, I could have attended the clinic or stayed locally for the tests and scans, which would have been infinitely easier.

The Ovidrel ovulation trigger injection was more ouchy than the Puregon, but it was also a bit exciting because it meant the big O was getting close and therefore potentially the creation of our baby! We were given an exact time for the trigger injection because it was directly tied in with the timing of Adam's ejaculation, and the insemination. For example, the first insemination was booked for 1pm 26/10/12. Consequently, Adam's sample collection was booked for 11:30am the same day and my ovulation trigger was to be injected at 8pm on 24/10/12.

Each of our IUI procedures were scheduled just after lunch so that we had time to make the trip to Canberra that morning. Before our appointment, we'd have lunch at marvellous café we discovered down the road from the clinic, so that was something special amongst the rigmarole. Another bonus was time spent with Adam in the car on our seven hour round trip. This was important at a time when we were feeling the strain as a couple. We had some rough times but upheld our promise to love one another in good times and in bad.

What struck me about the clinic was how stark and unfeeling it was. There were rows upon rows of brochures about the reproductive tract, infertility and assisted reproductive technologies. If I wanted medical information, it was there. But there was no warmth. There was nothing about the setting, the vibe or the information to offer comfort when I was feeling vulnerable and volatile.

The most critical part of insemination day was the role Adam had to play i.e. providing the swimmers. I was always of two minds how I felt about this. I felt for him that he had the pressure of 'performing' in a given time frame. It put him out of his comfort zone and, of course, he would've much preferred the traditional conception method. On the other hand I wished I could be so lucky that my one and only job (apart from managing hormonal Benita) was to provide a sample which was ultimately derived from pleasure with all the necessary supporting 'resources' provided in the room (aka the spank chamber). No probing, no gazillion needles, no one looking at his bits. Lucky bugger. His own private chamber to get the job done! We giggled the first time we saw it.

The room where the insemination took place was unremarkable and the 'bed' that was mine to lie on was small, cold and hard. How did above average sized people even fit on that bed? Lucky I was only average-sized. This was not the type of bed that I envisaged our future children being created on. The IUI procedure was not dissimilar to a pap smear, except the insemination apparatus was inserted further up – into the uterus – to deposit the sperm. It was over within a few minutes and generally with minor discomfort. Just another procedure with my legs apart for a total stranger, with my dignity slowly diminishing each time. It was important to me that we were together at the possible point of conception, so Adam sat up near my head and held my hand. For a man that was generally uncomfortable with 'girl stuff,' he handled the situation remarkably well. Once the sperm were where they should be, I stayed lying down with my knees bent for 10 minutes. After that we hoped for the best.

It gave me a whole new respect for those dear cows we inseminated.

The post-IUI treatment involved the use of vaginal progesterone pessaries (think oversized soft tablets) to keep my endometrium lush and support a possible pregnancy. Bleugh. I don't miss those messy horrid things that sent my hormones on a wild ride. I really felt their side effects, which for me was mostly mood swings and irritability.

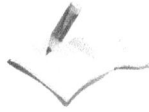

08/10/12 12:30pm
A letter to Adam (that I never gave him) [CYCLE 1]

Hi babe,

I hope you've had a good day and your meeting went well. The corn meat will be ready at 8:00 and I will be home about 9:00 unless the meeting is finished early. I'm walking out at 8:30 if it isn't done by then as it just goes too late!

Didn't want to call you and upset your day, so am writing this note in-stead. I also get very tired of hearing my voice in my head and out loud, so it's good to write this down to work out what to do about it. I have been really struggling today – on an absolute emotional rollercoaster. The same thing happened on Saturday afternoon when I sat down to work on my website. This morning I sat and stared at my computer screen before going to town, then went to town, felt a bit shaky, cried on the way home and then sat in my car for ½ hr crying and listening to music, which helped me feel a little better.

So, what's actually wrong, you say? Well, no doubt much of feeling this way is fuelled by hormones and anxiety (as much as I try to put it out of my mind) about our test results. It's difficult to explain how it feels to be in my body right now. One minute I feel good, in control, happy, yep I can do this. But then in the next breath, I want to yell, cry, and curl up in bed and block out the world. It's difficult to work normally and be chirpy and productive for clients while in this state.

It is an absolute mental battle right now of wanting to hide from people and not see anyone vs. forcing myself to be social. Why? Because I don't want them to ask me how I am, are we going to have children, what have I been up to, how am I feeling, etc. It's like talking about it gets it out of my head (which is a good thing) but at the same time…

(I didn't finish this letter and I can't recall exactly why. I think it was because I was getting analytical and bogged down and felt like I was getting nowhere with it).

11/10/12 [CYCLE 1]

I have so many thoughts whirling around in my head that I don't even know where to begin. Perhaps just beginning though is the most important. To free my mind from the swirling, whirling cloud that covers my mind and mixes all the thoughts together, and darkens them. You see, I'm in a dark place right now. I want to wallow here. But my inner strength is screaming at me, yelling from the sidelines 'get up, get going, we've gotta keep moving.' I want to let the darkness win for a little while, but I don't think it's in me. The sun has just come out and I feel lifted by that. Maybe it will help me see through the clouds hanging over my mind. I don't know.

I feel lost, like a nothing, like a massive void is in my body and any moment my mind is going to join in and jump into it, getting lost forever. I have always battled the darkness, that other side of me that's never content, never quite happy, always wanting more. Adam tells me to 'chill out' which is the best medicine I can ever take. He knows when I'm overthinking things, analysing, trying to 'work' everything out, making a mission of that. It's been happening a lot lately. My mind gets so full and confused, that I simply cannot think clearly. Any little thing, incident, that upsets my balance and controlled environment throws me for a mile, leaving me struggling to recover.

I wish I could find that easy-going, fun girl again. Where has she gone? She only comes out every now and then these days, and the rest of the time there's that worried, sad, serious woman trying, crucifying, analysing, not living, laughing and loving freely. Can I get her back?

Am I going to be strong enough to get through this?????????????????????? Living life in limbo, having no control over the process or the outcome, staying positive but not too hopeful, staying social but not too social, putting on a brave face and inwardly dying.

I am not happy; I am not striving for anything. I am just stopped. People say I need to learn how to just 'be' instead of 'doing' all the time, but I am happiest when I'm doing, achieving, learning, exploring, interacting, aiming. Is there anything wrong with that? Yes, I could be better at relaxing and the guilt trips I put myself on are not healthy.

I don't know what I want anymore. I don't know how to feel, how to be, what to focus on. My life feels dangerously unbalanced, spending far too much time on my own. But then at the moment I don't feel like being around other people much. I don't want to hear about babies; I don't want to hear about pregnancy. I don't want to talk about doctors. I don't want to explain how I'm feeling (it changes so often). I don't want to hear people's stories and remedies. I just want the world to go away, but then again it helps for me to talk about some things, to some people. See what I mean about confused.

Maybe I have lost my ability to cope with life. Maybe I have become fragile, like a glass doll, that can go alright when things are going her way, but when things change or get tough, she breaks. Maybe I need to really work a lot harder at being content and accepting. I go okay at this in short bursts, but then I get off track. Why can't I stick to it? I sometimes feel like I can't commit to anything – is that because I am always wanting to be in control of every situation? Probably.

. . .

When I wrote the above journal entry on the eleventh of October 2012, I was sitting on the couch drinking a bottle of red wine in the middle of the day. I had made *the* phone call to the fertility clinic to find out my Cycle 1 +14 (14 days post insemination) hCG level was 0. I had been instructed to have the blood test on +14 because the +12 hCG level teetered out to be <5 which meant we needed to monitor whether it would go up or down. It went down as far as it can go – a big fat zero. Not even a trace of pregnancy hormone.

Infertility is defined as the inability to conceive a pregnancy after 12 months of unprotected sexual intercourse. We were officially infertile. Or I was officially infertile. I didn't know which. We were now a statistic.

It was an obliterating blow to acknowledge that even when the sperm was put where it needed to go at exactly the right time, I STILL didn't conceive. My self-esteem and faith in my body really took a hit and this was a turning point for me in terms of my mental health. The bottle of red wine was not normal for me, it was a knee-jerk method of escapism, to escape the gaping void I described in my journal. To numb the pain and frustration.

I see now that I had been gradually and inaudibly slipping down the treacherous slope toward mental illness for a while. I had been pushing on and pushing through, but I wasn't addressing the steady decline in my state of mind. My thoughts were jumbled, there was no order to my mind. I knew I wasn't right and had a general feeling of unease, but I didn't know what to do about it and thought it would sort itself out. I kept telling myself to make the best of the situation I was in and hang in there because surely, we would fall pregnant soon, which would solve the problem.

I had conquered numerous 'hard-to-achieve' things in my life: a University medal, leadership awards, winning Queensland Rural Ambassador in 2007, a successful business, buying a house and farm, to name a few. I was a guru at trying hard for success. I knew how to play the game. But not this bloody trying game in which trying hard felt futile. What I needed was some professional help, but I didn't reach out for it.

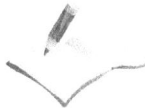

14/10/12 10:39pm [CYCLE 2]

Back from two nights away at Batemans Bay in celebration of our 2nd wedding anniversary, and also to have some quiet time together before windrowing and harvest starts. It was also an escape from reality, from the strain of fertility treatment and just real life stuff. Its day 2 today and I started my injections again. We found out last week that cycle 1 was unsuccessful, which was a huge disappointment, and really hard to take that news. I was a bit of a wreck last week due to that. It's like an emotional rollercoaster and sometimes I just want to jump off the ride. Sometimes the ride de-rails and sometimes it's on track, but pretty much all the time it travels the highs and the lows. I feel stronger today and ready to tackle cycle 2. I have the positive words and thought processes at the ready to employ this week. Well, I have started to feel very tired all of a sudden…time for sleep and up in the morning to go for a run to burn off some of the holiday cheer! We had such a lovely time! Night. B xo

7/11/12 [CYCLE 2]

Today I feel like I could give it all up. It's just too hard and I am so tired of this merry go round of emotions every month. I do such a good job of holding myself up for the first 2/3 of the month, only to let myself become vulnerable and hopeful close to the results date based on the latest pregnancy symptom I have, and then fall flat on my face.

09/11/12 [CYCLE 2]

It's amazing how a bit of sleep and some time in the sunshine can help your perspective. In the last few days we have learned that our 2nd fertility treatment cycle (medicated OI & IUI) was unsuccessful. As it is any month when trying to conceive, this was hard news to take. Together with a head cold and 600mg of progesterone pessaries per day, I haven't had the best few days. I'm tired, depressed and so angry (a side effect of pessaries, I find). Spending the day with Ad checking for pests in the canola oilseed crops.

. . .

There was a novelty factor associated with Cycle 1 because it was new and I felt empowered being on a new path. Fronting up for Cycle 2 felt very different – it had a rougher edge to it that I worried was going to take a chunk out of me. By the time Cycle 3 came around I was a mess. The whole process was fraught with emotion.

Everything felt hard and hopeless. I was alone and in my head too much. I had the support of my beautiful friends and family on tap, but I didn't know how to share in words what I was experiencing. What could anyone do anyway? One particular day I drove to the property where Adam was working because I wasn't coping well and needed a chat. He was in the middle of working with his harvest team and so was understandably busy but the encounter ended with me unfairly yelling at him and making him feel guilty that he wasn't helping me. He didn't know how and neither did I. I swayed about all over the place and the unease morphed into anxiety and depression.

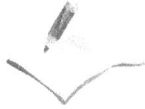

13/11/12 11:19pm [CYCLE 3]

Harvest is in full swing here with 9 CASE headers out there in the darkness, harvesting canola, with chaser bins buzzing around them like bees. Adam is on one of the headers tonight, doing night shift for one of the older gentlemen who can't (or doesn't like to) work at night. I completed my 4th day of harvest catering today... phew. 2 meals per day + snacks, for 20 men, for 3 weeks...I must be mad! I wanted to challenge myself and do something different other than sit in front of a computer screen. It's paid work and should be quite profitable for us. I'm enjoying it so far, though it's a lot of work. It's not just the cooking; it's the washing up and shopping/ordering on top of the cooking, that adds up. Anyway, no doubt, I will get better at it as the weeks roll on! It's bedtime now, Goodnight. B xo

21/11/12 [CYCLE 3]

I had a meltdown today. Today is Day 11 of our third OI/IUI cycle. Holding it all together, going well, doing fine, yes, I'm good, hanging in there, and then whammo; today it all came crashing down. I woke up tired, organised what I needed to before leaving home for Wagga Wagga, and then left late (great). With an almost 2hr drive to get where I needed to go, I rang the ultrasound clinic at 9:20am to let them know

I was going to be about 10mins late for my 9:30am appointment. "Oh, but your appointment is at 9am so you're already 20 mins late," came the voice through the phone. Bullshit – my appointment is definitely at 9:30, I wrote it down yesterday, I thought. The smallest thing, that's all it took to get me in the wrong frame of mind for the day. I just said I'd be there as soon as I could. I knew that if one of the receptionists questioned me, I'd break down on the spot, so I just concentrated on smiling sweetly and pretending nothing was wrong. Luckily, when I did get there, the staff were great and I almost went straight in (5 blissful minutes reading Fifty Shades Freed in the waiting room) and for the first time in my whole gynaecological experience in the last six years, I had a male sonographer. Oh my God, don't panic. It was fine – he was very professional and kind. A few follicles on the left ovary and a handful on the right, though it took him a long time to ascertain this, which does nothing for one's confidence in said sonographer's ability. Anyhow, once that was over, I headed to the blood collection centre down the road for D11 blood test. They drew a vial first go which was much better than my last blood test two days ago (two goes) and the one before that (three goes). Following that I headed to Gloria Jeans for a coffee and to keep reading Fifty Shades Freed (addicted). See here lays the problem – I would never normally do this on a work day. At the moment I simply feel like everything is too hard and I don't want to care about anything. So... in the end I sat for... 4 hours... reading – first in Gloria Jeans, then outside Gloria Jeans on a bench, then in my car (by this time with a sandwich and bottle of water). That book is so bloody good but that's not the point, I was avoiding facing real life. Today, I just could not cope with real life – emails, phone calls, work, shopping and jobs while in Wagga. I finished the book in the back seat of my car. Then I sat there for a moment unable to think, make a decision, do anything, and then rang my Mum. For an hour I cried, poured my heart out and told Mum things about how I'm feeling that I haven't really admitted to anyone, probably even myself, in an articulated way. By the end of it, I was exhausted but it felt good to have emptied some of the burden in my brain and my heart. Did I solve anything? Yes, I did. The major thing, I think at the root of how I'm feeling about everything at the moment – having a baby, my work, my life – is that I feel like a failure. How can I not fulfil the most basic purpose of human existence, to reproduce? How can my body betray me this way? WHAT IS WRONG IN THERE?

There must be something wrong. How is it that we can try, do every-thing right, do everything in our power, do our absolute best, for TWO YEARS and still not succeed in producing a healthy, viable embryo that wants to implant and stay in my uterus? Over time these feelings of deteriorating self-confidence and depletion of my core essence as a woman, have started to radiate into other parts of my life, until I simply just feel... lost. All my life I have been able to achieve whatever I set my mind to, but now, this one thing that I want more than anything in the world, it eludes me, taunts me, month after month. And. It. Is. Driving. Me. Crazy. Somehow, somehow, I have to get through this, yet I have very little hope for this month's cycle and just don't know if I can cope with the disappointment of another negative result. That little voice inside me says 'yes you can' and I know that I'll handle it, whatever is thrown at me, but at what cost? Matters are not helped with yesterday being 12 months since we lost Ronnie Bean. Yesterday it made me smile, and cry, to see the lemon tree (aptly named Ronnie) starting to bear its first fruit – tiny little green lemons that with some TLC will flourish. I hoped none of the harvest workers were here watching me while I stood stroking a little lemon, the reminder I have of our baby. I will never get past that horrible memory of losing our baby in the hospital. I think, after today's events, I should just go to bed.

. . .

Cycle 2 was unsuccessful and Cycle 3 ended up being cancelled as a result of my follicles not responding well enough to the drugs. It was not worth paying the fee for the cycle and going ahead with the insemination as there was no dominant follicle from which an egg could be released. They instructed Adam and I to try naturally instead for the month. In a robotic manner I still underwent six blood tests and two ultrasound scans in the space of 16 days, along with progesterone pessaries until +10 when the blood test revealed I wasn't pregnant. Well, actually, on that day it showed my hCG was <5 but not 0, so I was supposed to go the next day for another test. I didn't. I was so done with it all and held absolutely zilch hope. I had failed.

In some ways I was relieved that Cycle 3 didn't go ahead because I was so far removed from a healthy mindset and I didn't want to be pregnant in that state. I didn't care anymore. I hit rock bottom on the twenty-first of November and was in a black hole of despair in mind and spirit. Not physically though – I was still high functioning from the outside looking in. There was rarely any lying around or an inability to get up and face the day. I was going through the motions of life and pushing myself immensely by singlehandedly catering for Adam's harvest crew. But on the inside – it was chaos. For me the black hole presents itself as mental paralysis, confusion and a sense of hopelessness.

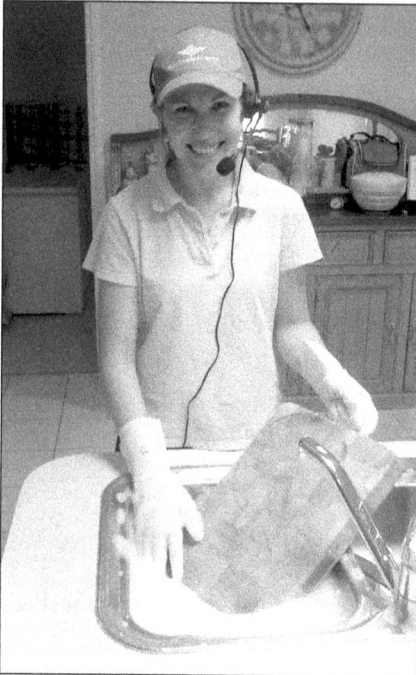

Multitasking and putting on a brave face catering for Adam's harvest crew, but inwardly dying, Back Creek November 2012.

Amongst the darkness there was one ray of sunshine in the form of a Sydney business coach I sought out mid-October to help me find my way with Sunburnt Country. I was doing the work, but at a strategic level I was stale and aimless. For a long time, I had wanted coaching but I delayed it assuming it was too expensive. When I became desperate for support, I didn't care what the cost was – I was going to do it. My heart pounded as I contacted Robert. I didn't think a city coach would be interested in working with little old me out in the big wheat paddock with my small business. Thankfully, I was mistaken. The coaching I received from him saved me and my business. I felt a spark of excitement at a deeper level that I hadn't felt since closing our Gunnedah office. I got flashes of how I felt when first creating Sunburnt Country five years before – a creative mindset rather than a disintegrating one. It got me back in the game and gave me something to look forward to for the year ahead other than TTC.

I knew what I needed after the previous three months of struggle: my family, my home and a clean break from all of it.

Early in December I drove north to Kylee and Anthony's property in Queensland for cattle mustering and niece and nephew cuddles, and then went another four hours northeast to my parents at the home farm for an early family Christmas celebration. After a few weeks of R&R, I was beginning to feel like myself again and I was happy to head south to join Adam and the Bensch's for Christmas.

**For detailed medical notes from these OI & IUI cycles please see the Appendix.

A special note on trying not to cry

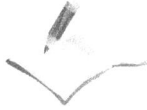

27/10/12

It's official, I hate baby showers. It's not that I don't like the concept of baby showers, because I agree that impending baby arrivals are a thing to celebrate; I just don't like the awkwardness of them and the stupid games! I even won two of the games at the shower I attended today and that still didn't make it any better. Second to the games (and only beaten by a whisker) is present opening time. I do not enjoy sitting around oohing and aahing over baby gifts, listening to women apologising because their gift is 'practical.' It was tough for me to attend the baby shower today. I am delighted for my friend and I wanted to be there for her, but on the inside I was doing my utmost not to relate everything to our situation and burst into tears. When you're at a point in time where you're avoiding the 'baby conversation' in public, particularly with random strangers, baby showers are obviously going to be a challenge. Perhaps I'll feel differently about baby showers when I'm pregnant.

Baby news, baby showers, christenings and first birthday parties were coming thick and fast at this point in life as many of our fellow 30-ish friends were also in the trying years. There were times it felt like we were the only ones trying while they were all succeeding!

It was tough not being in their club yet; being happy for them whilst growing increasingly bitter and unhappy about our own situation. I beat myself up about it a lot. I wanted to genuinely share in their joy, but sometimes I didn't genuinely feel it. I hope it didn't show on the outside, as I never wanted to let our challenges impact someone else's happiness.

A few examples stick in my mind:

I went to the first birthday party of the son of a good friend and it took every ounce of my strength not to cry and run away. I almost didn't go in the first place. I made a feeble excuse and left early. I thought my friend would get it without me having to explain, but she was oblivious. And so should she be – it was a special day for their family.

Adam's younger brother Ryan rang to share the beautiful news that they were expecting; my sister-in-law was 15 weeks pregnant. He didn't say so, but they'd been putting off telling us because they knew we were having a hard time. Of course, I was overjoyed for them, and sent my congratulations, but first I cried. Why couldn't that be us? That was my common reaction during those years as we continued to hear more pregnancy and baby announcements.

It was a double-edged sword – the wanting your family and friends to share their news with you and not treat you differently, but at the same time not wanting to know. I was grateful for their sensitivity and compassion, yet disappointed if they didn't tell me they were pregnant. It was tricky! It was a blessing to be able to hide behind carefully constructed text messages and take myself off social media.

When I was in a good frame of mind other people's stories wouldn't affect me too much. Other times I couldn't handle it. My feelings were a potent cocktail of frustration, grief and fear – of what had happened, what hadn't yet happened, and what might never happen. Whether I felt positive or negative (or somewhere in between) changed daily; sometimes momentarily!

Even when I felt strong, holding a baby and looking down upon him/her tested my resolve to its limit. I had to remain as emotionally detached as I could, otherwise I would've ended up a blubbering mess.

The saying 'what you focus on, you attract' seemed so true during this period. I felt like I was attracting every pregnant woman in Australia to walk down the street when I did. All I could see were bellies and prams. I disliked feeling this way as I prefer to be happy for others, not loathing them. I just wanted it so badly for myself too.

At what point is it okay to hide away and avoid the baby showers, christenings and parties for the sake of self-preservation? I pondered that. There were some occasions I didn't attend, but mostly I pulled up my big girl undies, swallowed, held down the cocktail and smiled my way through it.

How many people do you tell what you're going through? What do you tell them? You want them to know so that they understand, but then things change once they do know. They don't readily talk to you about pregnancy and babies, they don't know what to say, they don't know if you want to be left alone or supported. Then you're adding another person to the list of people waiting to hear if you're pregnant. Sometimes it's easier not to involve them for those reasons… which leaves you feeling even more alone.

Our families and a few close friends were in our inner circle of knowing, but as a general rule I hid away when I could. It was simpler that way.

When random unaware people asked, "When are you going to have a baby?" through held-back tears I would say, "We're trying." And that futile feeling would surface.

I think it's time we replace the 'we're trying' expression with something more positive and conducive to conception, minus the trying connotation. If someone asks "When are you going to have a baby?" I encourage you to replace "We're trying" with one of the below suggestions and notice the difference it makes in your body. To me these alternatives feel expanded rather than contracted. If the person asking you the question looks at you like you're a bit crazy well that's their business, this is about you and creating a desirable mindset.

"Our baby is on its way to me."

"I'm looking forward to conceiving."

"I'm preparing to conceive."

"We are conceiving."

"I expect to conceive any day now."

"I'm ready to conceive and receive."

Have fun with this!

CHAPTER 7

Trying to let go

I emerged into the sunlight, squinting, as I clambered up and over the ledge of the black hole. I lay there for a time, adjusting to nature's elements that I'd been devoid of. I'd been here before. I knew I was going to make it now. I wasn't lost forever. I was still me. Thank God, I was still me. I was going to smile again.

I stood slowly, dusted myself off and circulated a few lungfuls of fresh air. I felt lighter, free, stronger. Where to now? We continue to receive a lesson until we learn it and evidently, I still hadn't mastered the lesson of catching myself before the freefall. But back on my feet and with a clearer mind I had the opportunity to start anew, and for that I was thankful.

I couldn't control this thing. I had tried hard and lost. I had been hanging on so tightly, doing all I could to make it happen and in the end I still landed with a thud. For something to change I had to change something – starting within me.

It was January 2013. I started to focus on letting go of the expectations, timeframes and ideals I held about starting a family. I didn't abandon them, but I strove to release my vice-like grip. The black hole forced this – I knew that it was imperative for my survival. I *had* to let go a bit. I deliberately became more aware of my limiting thoughts. I wanted to slow and catch my thoughts so that when they were unhelpful, I could flip them. I adopted the mantra "whatever happens I will be okay" and when a thought or feeling cropped up that wasn't helpful, I told myself to "let it go." This played on repeat. "Let it go" was soothing to me and I imagined the unhelpful stuff floating away into the universe. I was far from Zen-like, it was trial and error and messy, as navigating a new path usually is. I was healing from the inside out which takes time, persistence and a gentleness with oneself.

It was still scary not knowing if, when and how we would achieve our goal. Looking out from the ledge there stretched an open expanse with no known end or landmarks in sight. How long? How far? What will happen along the way? I didn't want it any less and we never stopped trying to conceive, but my mindset around it became more healthy and accepting. The constricting sense of utter desperation was gone. In hindsight I was appreciative of the black hole because on the other side of it came new awareness and personal growth. All I could do was put one foot in front of the other, keep trying and focus on the things I could control.

Everything was soon going to change dramatically once again.

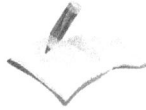

14/01/13

Almost two months after my Wagga Wagga meltdown I am feeling much stronger and happier about life. I owe this to having some lovely time with Adam (harvest finished before Christmas) and our families prior to and over the Christmas period, particularly my family in Queensland. Having a break from work and treatment since the first week in December has also been wonderful. I feel like I have so much time not having to plan my life around blood tests, scans and my moods; it's been great! Yet today I started to get that feeling nagging at me, that mixture of frustration and sadness, that 'why me' thought alongside the images of me pregnant or holding a child, that I long for in real life. I think I was so ready for a break that I was relieved not to think about it anymore, and then I was so distracted by other events going on in our lives that today was the first time I'd allowed myself to think about the trying game again. This past month we have been pretending not to try – that whole game of blocking it from my mind, yet secretly hoping we might be pregnant by natural means. Wouldn't that be heaven! Unfortunately, it's not the case as I have just finished my period.

Adam and I came to another critical crossroad in our lives sooner than we anticipated and the rollout of our five-year plan in the south came to a screeching halt. Things were not working out with Adam's job as we'd hoped. A new farming opportunity with my family beckoned in Queensland, so relatively suddenly we decided we would relocate in March to Goondiwindi – a small but thriving country town on the border between NSW and Qld. It was a complete role reversal for Adam and I, now to be heading away from his family and toward mine. It was hard for him, and tough for the Bensch family to accept, but once more we were doing what we thought best for us (and our imaginary future family) in the long term.

This also helped my state of mind, planning to be heading north again. Our time at Back Creek had been rocky for me, to say the least. I welcomed the new start in a town we had long been fond of, closer to my family, working together towards our next farming dream. Adam's new agchemical sales manager job would allow us to see each other more often, and new Sunburnt Country business opportunities were presenting themselves.

Our decision to move raised the questions: what's next with our trying, and where will we have our fertility treatment? We didn't feel like it was a good fit for us to continue at the Canberra clinic where we had our OI/IUI cycles. We were ready to look at other options. To be truthful I never wanted to go back there again. Of course, it wasn't their fault that our cycles were unsuccessful, however I didn't connect with the energy of that clinic. Good riddance, yukky nothing-ness clinic of bad memories.

Geographically the closest specialists to Goondiwindi were in Toowoomba or Brisbane, but two friends of mine had recommended a reputable and very nice fertility and IVF specialist based at Genea, Sydney. He regularly consulted in Tamworth, which was only a few hours from our new home. Dr. Mark Livingstone is his name. Our approach was that if we were going to do this, we were going to do it with the best... even at the sake of convenience. Once we moved to Goondiwindi it was a 750km/nine hour drive one way to Sydney by car. From what we could tell, Dr. Livingstone was up there with the best. The fact that he travelled to a regional location to make his services accessible to country people also told us of his nature and was a big tick for us. Yay, another decision made – we would arrange a meeting soon.

For a while a family member had been recommending a tarot card reader in Wagga Wagga who had read her cards and how interesting (and freakishly accurate) the experience proved to be. I was curious, but too frightened about what I might find out to go ahead with it. But with our move looming curiosity got the better of me and I decided it was now or never. So, I made an appointment, pushed down my nerves and showed up to have my cards read. I was astounded with what was uncovered, and strangely it was another turning point for me in coping with the trying rollercoaster ride.

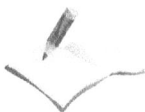

01/02/13

It is Friday evening and I am enjoying a glass of cold white wine... mmm. No, I'm still not pregnant. Normal not-trying type people would not know or appreciate this, but we of the trying type consider every month whether the alcoholic drink we're enjoying will be our last. I have now been in this state of mind for over two years. I reckon a psychologist would have something to say about it. Today is Day 25 of my cycle (another thing non-trying folk wouldn't think about) and perhaps I shouldn't even be having this drink 'just in case.' I have been through a lot of 'just in case' months and ended up disappointed so I have decided to keep living my life during the two week wait (2WW). As Adam tells me, I end up more stressed by worrying about what I should and shouldn't do during the 2WW, which can't be better than being my normal self.

The last few weeks have been very... interesting. Within our family and friends, we've had a new baby born, a pregnancy announced, a family friend pass away and everything in between, or so it feels like. The circle of life at its best. I also had one of the most astonishing experiences of my life – I had my tarot cards read for the first time. It's not something I ever really believed or was interested in, but after having it done it has changed my mind. Among many, many other things that were revealed to me I learned that (according to my reader) I will be a mother... gulp... to 3 children. I have the recording to prove it and I'm sticking to it!

Apparently, we'll have 2 children – twins or born close together – and then a bit later, a baby boy. I don't know whether it will be true and I'm not going to treat it as gospel, but it was certainly nice to hear something so reassuring. I guess we'll have to wait and see!

. . .

Three children she predicted! Three! She was certain I'd become a mother and she reassured me we were making the right life choices. It's like a switch was flicked having my cards read. Something changed in me. It was a bit out there, but her accuracy regarding other areas of my life was so spot on that it was hard not to buy into her predictions. I was breathing fast as I sat in the car afterwards, replaying her words, a wetness in my eyes. She says this is going to happen… just imagine! Then and there I gave myself permission to place my faith in a higher power. What did I have to lose? She gave me the gift of hope.

Hope. The mighty four letter word in the TTC journey.

It had been hard to remain hopeful at times when the disappointment was inexorable, but I realised there was always hope, and for us – still so much hope. We would get there one way or another. "What about adoption?" I heard from a few people. I'd thought of it too, frequently, and researched it, but I was offended at the suggestion of it from others. Didn't they think we could achieve this? How could they offhandedly propose something so significant? My clipped reply was, "we're a long way from that." There were still many avenues for Adam and I yet to explore.

Amid the packing and planning we met with Dr. Livingstone and his Scottish accent in Sydney at the end of February. The aim of the visit was to discuss the next steps in our assisted conception journey. At the conclusion of the consultation the options presented to us were:

1) Start IVF straight away
2) Have a laparoscopy and hysteroscopy to diagnose and treat any issues such as endometriosis, try to conceive naturally for a few months and then start IVF

Another decision to make. We decided before we left the Sydney CBD; possibly even before we left Dr. Livingstone's office. It seemed like the more sensible approach to check and make sure everything was alright before starting IVF. We wanted the peace of mind that we were giving IVF our best shot without the interference of endometriosis or other unseen issues. It meant waiting longer (I was getting better at that) and a potentially unnecessary surgery, but could sidestep further cost and heartbreak in the long run. I knew what to expect of the surgery and recovery, and was curious to know what state my endometriosis was in compared to 2007. We let the receptionist know we chose option two and waited to be advised of a surgery date.

We had the choice of the fourteenth of March or fifteenth of April. The sooner the better from my perspective, so although fourteen March would only be a few days after relocating to Goondiwindi, we went with that. Not typical at all for Benita to pack everything in and make life as complicated as possible.

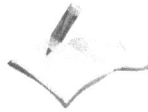

20/03/13

This time last week (Qld time) we were driving through Sydney on our way to my friend Mandy's house to stay the night before my surgery at 7am the next morning, Thursday 14 March. It was a late arrival due to our late departure from Goondiwindi. We hadn't known until 10am the morning we were supposed to leave that my surgery was definitely going ahead. My period was 3 days late (due to the stress of moving, I think) and didn't arrive until the wee hours of Wednesday, so I wasn't sure if the surgery could go ahead. I even had to have a blood test on Tuesday for a possible early pregnancy, which unfortunately wasn't the case. Talk about stressful! Anyhow, we were pleased the surgery went ahead as scheduled. The outcome of the surgery was the diagnosis of mild endometriosis, which didn't come as a surprise. All else in my reproductive tract was normal, for which we're very grateful. It's all relative really isn't it? Someone like my older sister – who conceived naturally so easily and has three gorgeous healthy children – probably thinks, "you poor thing" for all that we've gone through. Then I think about other women who have conditions far worse than mine, or couples who jointly have terrible troubles and I think, "you poor things." I feel so lucky in comparison because we still have hope... and time on our side. So here I am a week later, stitches out, tummy not so bloated and sore, chest not so painful from the gas. My energy levels are up and I'm bouncing back from the procedure. I spoke to Dr. Livingstone today and we have made a plan to start IVF in June. Prior to that we are to meet with our Nurse Coordinator and Adam needs to have a fancy pants Genea semen analysis which will require another trip to Sydney. I think this time we'll look into flying! That 9 hour drive to and from Sydney will do me for a while.

How am I feeling about all this? I would say I've been sufficiently distracted for the past few months. Now here we are in our new house, in a new town with a new life at our feet. It still feels quite surreal. As we get to know people here, I know I'll be confronted with the typical question: "do you have children?" To which I reply, "not yet," as though I hold all the power in the world to decide when we'll bear offspring. Ha! If only they knew! I guess things will fall into place. In other exciting developments I have signed up for a 12-week body transformation which starts soon. My goal is to lose 3-4kg, tone up and increase my fitness. I'm not happy with my body shape at the moment and I think this is the most unfit I've been in a long, long time. I'm keen to change this and be as healthy as I can be during the next few months. Oh my gosh, I can't believe we're going to do IVF. Who would have thought the IVF story would be mine?

· · ·

We knew we had entered a new league as soon as we stepped foot in the Genea building in the heart of Sydney. And we knew we had made the right decision to go there. It was next level in expertise, professionalism and service, and a more holistic approach, which I really liked. Due to our science backgrounds, Adam and I also liked the focus on cutting-edge research and technology. Dr. Livingstone was delightful and I felt very comfortable with him (and could listen to him all day).

We reverted back to the good old au naturelle trying naturally stage between my surgery recovery and waiting to start IVF. It was an unusual time. If we didn't become pregnant naturally, we were going to do IVF, so the pressure was kind of off. BUT if we did conceive, we'd avoid the intrusion and cost of IVF all together, so in that sense there was pressure. It felt like our last-ditch effort to see if we could tick the box on our own.

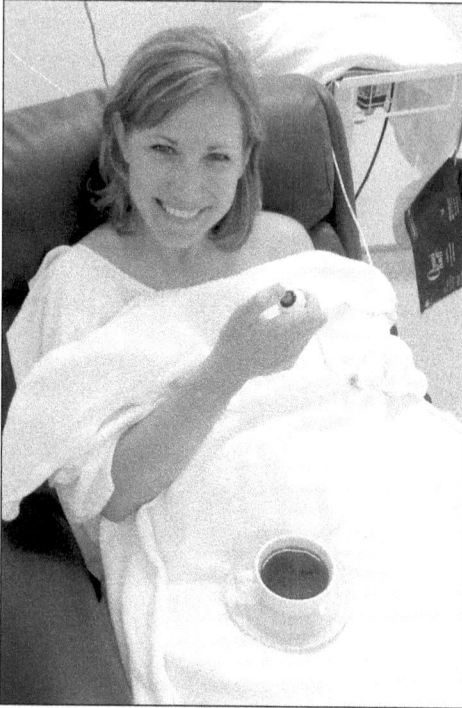

Recovering from my second laparoscopy and hysteroscopy, Sydney March 2013.

Dr. Livingstone counselled that we should have intercourse every second day around the middle of my cycle, which we did. Making love was still a different kettle of fish when doing it because you 'should,' and when preoccupied with optimising the sperm's journey with positions, legs up, legs down, positive thoughts, all layered with the question "is this going to be the time *it* happens?" Honestly, does any of that stuff make a difference? People get pregnant in any manner of situations despite their best intentions not to so I really did wonder how us perfectly orchestrating the missionary position would be the one thing that got us over the line. But we did it anyway, just in case.

When not unpacking or in the missionary position, I was working and enjoying the pleasures of living in town, like being able to walk to the bakery for fresh bread and a real coffee. With the help of my business coach, I unearthed a new calling – coaching. I started studying to become a coach and incorporate business coaching into my services. I was overjoyed to be learning and working towards a goal again. I wanted to phase in coaching and gradually phase out some of the marketing services I had offered for many years. I loved the collaborative nature of the coaching relationship and how I could empower, encourage and support others to make important life-giving and life-changing choices. To wholeheartedly step into this role, first I had to do the work on myself, and continue to show up for myself. With restored vision and energy, I set about re-creating Sunburnt Country, and more importantly, myself.

My mental and emotional health was the best it had been in a very long time, and I hoped that would be listed on the positive side of the conceiving ledger. I sincerely wondered if over the past few years God (or someone/something) had been out to teach me a lesson in patience, acceptance and understanding what's most important in life – looking after yourself and those nearest and dearest to you. Perhaps so.

We made our plans to travel to Genea for Adam's final andrology test, our nurse coordinator interview and a counselling appointment, all as a precursor to starting IVF. Our appointments were booked for the twentieth of May. It felt great to have that sorted and on the calendar, but making the appointments and dipping myself back in that treatment world for a few hours did have an impact on me. Deep breath. I had to be brave and strong to move forward.

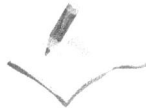

11/05/13

I cannot believe it's the eleventh day of May already. In fact, the eleventh day of May is a few hours from being over. This time next week we'll be in a Brisbane motel readying ourselves for our flight to Sydney the following morning. Once again, I'm waiting for my period to arrive… and the typical signs are starting to show.

We left Genea on the afternoon of the twentieth of May, weary, overwhelmed with information and clutching a grass green insulated carry bag containing the medical supplies I would need for our first IVF cycle. It could easily have been mistaken for a bag you'd take your lunch in to work. There was nothing on it to identify it for what it was. I imagined an army of people, like ants, every day marching away from the Genea nest holding their green lunch boxes full of drugs and needles, hopes and dreams. The following week we learnt that both Adam's and my suite of test results were all favourable. There were no more hoops to jump through – we were all set.

In early June family and friends joined us for a surprise party that I organised for Adam's 30th birthday. It was rare to have both sides of our family together at one time, so it was a special night for us and the succeeding week with visiting family was lots of fun. It was the last 'normal' week for us before starting IVF, so I was pleased to be distracted by Adam's birthday, the State of Origin rugby league game (eight years on from the bet Adam and I made when we first met) and a trip to Brisbane to watch the Queensland Reds vs British Lions rugby union match.

I was scared about starting IVF as it meant going back to that place in my mind and heart where I hadn't been for most of the year. Somehow, I needed to maintain the strong, happy state of mind I was in. There were so many questions and fears: how will I feel, will it work, what results will we get, how soon can we afford to do another cycle, how much will it hurt…? I was as scared of success as I was of failure. But I was terrified of trying really hard and failing again. Over and over I whispered, "Let it go Benita, let it go."

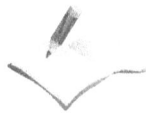

12/06/13

As soon as my period comes we'll be starting our first IVF cycle. Today is Day 30 and I wonder when my old friend will arrive. Isn't it ironic the love-hate relationship we develop with our menstrual cycle when TTC? Most months it breaks my heart when she arrives and I spend the best part of the day picking up the pieces to stay hopeful for another month. This month it's the opposite – I am willing her to arrive. Her arrival signals a new chapter in our journey, the green light telling us we can GO and get on with it, after talking about it and thinking about it for so long. I am scared about this new chapter, I admit it, but at the same time it means we're another step closer to our ultimate goal. A goal that's felt so elusive, but may be achieved in a matter of weeks. Only time will tell. I have been feeling anxious and angry this past week. My poor darling Adam has copped the brunt of it. SO ANGRY and these last few days I have been asking myself why. Angry at what? Angry because I feel I've been dealt a tough hand? Angry because we have to go through this? Angry at Adam because he can't do this for me? Angry at Adam because he's not giving this as much attention as I think he should? Angry that I'll have to stop doing the 12WBT (which I've been doing for the past 5 weeks and have lost 2.3kg so far – yippee!). Angry at all those people who I know are going to say things to me that will make me even angrier? Angry that my world is being interrupted for two weeks to go through the processes and procedures that are involved? Angry because I've walked this path before (to a lesser degree) and I know how I might feel? Angry to potentially step back into the black hole that consumed me at the end of last year? Maybe all of the above. Maybe I'm mistaking anger for fear. Today I had a good talk with both Kylee and my Mum. I am so blessed to have an amazing family and particularly two amazing sisters and a mother that I am very close to. Kylee and I had a cry today when she gave me my birthday card followed by a few truths that I probably needed to hear, like to stop being hard on myself, to put faith in myself and to think of this experience as the beginning of my journey with our child. Wow. Thanks Ky, you are incredibly special and wise.

. . .

The beginning of my journey with our child, she said. That left a big impression on me. I hadn't thought of it like that. It shifted my perspective toward this being a co-creative journey; that maybe as I was working my way towards him/her, he/she was also making his/her way towards me. That we're in it together, that I was already a Mum in spirit, all we needed was to bring about the physical form. The words 'our child' also plucked me out of the depths of my focus on the *how*, and reminded me of the *why* we were doing this.

Gulp.   Here   we   go.

A special note on time

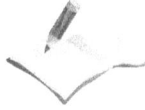

01/02/13

I used to be so conscious of my biological clock I could almost hear it ticking in my brain. I am 31 years of age. In 4.5 months I'll be 32. Shit.

. . .

We comment a lot about time in everyday life: how it goes slowly, how it flies, how time stands still, how we don't have enough time, or wish we had more time. Time felt like my biggest enemy during our trying journey. I butted heads and wrestled with it, I felt like I was pushing against it and it was pushing back at me. I expended so much energy thinking and stressing about time, which is ludicrous because it's one of the only constants in our life!

I now know that *time* wasn't my enemy, it was my *perception* of it, and *attitude* towards it that was the problem. I now know that my greatest challenge was actually managing the woman in the mirror.

Each day we are given the gift of 86,400 seconds. We can't change or manage time, all we can do is choose how we wish to invest that gift through our activities which stem from our thoughts. And we have the power to control our thoughts.

Instead of worrying about time ticking away, the implications of aging, and that not being what I wanted, I could have redirected that energy into using my thoughts to build and hold the picture of what I *did* want, not what I *didn't*. I didn't have that awareness then. There was no changing the fact that I was getting older, but I wish I had known how to be in flow with it rather than raging against it.

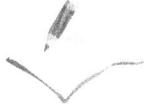

06/06/13

In 13 days I will be 32. Once upon a time, if someone had told me I still wouldn't be a mother at 32, I would have laughed in their face. I would not have thought it possible because it wasn't part of my grand plan. Now I'm staring down the barrel of being 33 when we have our first child and I must accept that it's the way it's going to be. I know that really it's not that old, or too old, but it's older than expected and it has ramifications. That said, in the past 12 months I have done my best to stop putting pressure on myself and setting expectations and timeframes around falling pregnant. I had to, to keep myself going.

. . .

I have learnt that the most joyful times in my life appear when flow replaces struggle. Flow feels… easy. And graceful, peaceful, and productive. There is flow when things happen in life when and how they are meant to – at the right time. I love being in the flow. For a long time I most certainly wasn't, but as I learnt to let go, things were in flow a bit more often and I felt… better.

CHAPTER 8

Trying with IVF

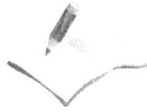

13/06/13 CYCLE DAY 31 -> CYCLE DAY 1 - Thursday

My period is due to arrive today. I've been worried and anxious all week about when it will come... will it be late, will I be able to have a blood test, etc. I need not have worried as my period pain started with ferocity at 5am which led to Panadol and broken sleep until 8:30am. With relief, I called Genea at 8:45 to tell them today is DAY 1. By the time they returned my call I'd taken myself off for my blood test. Fingers, toes, everything crossed that the results will be fine and all can go ahead. All of our plans for this month hinge on it (along with my emotions). Ad is away so the waiting rests with me.

. . .

I waited with bated breath until about 1pm on Friday the fourteenth of June 2013 for Genea to call me back with my blood test result from the previous day. "Your results are good," they said. I didn't know exactly what they meant, but they followed it with "you can go ahead with IVF this month." I took a deep breath, and mumbled, "Ok, thank you." I felt like the weight of the world had been lifted off my shoulders. It was finally happening. At 1:30pm I injected my first daily dose of Puregon into my tummy. It was like reuniting with a familiar but annoying acquaintance. What comforted me was that we had a common goal at least.

I'd learnt some logistical lessons from our OI/IUI days and was looking for the least stress option. I surmised that as the middle of my cycle neared, it would be wise to stay in a city where I could have the required blood tests and scans, and the results to Sydney when they were needed. We decided the major regional centre of Tamworth in northern NSW was the best choice. Subsequently, I had booked a farm cottage in the Bendemeer area 45 minutes from Tamworth. It was more economical than staying in town, with the added benefit of rural serenity. It was also my way of hiding away. I didn't feel like being in town where I'd likely run into someone I knew and have to explain why I was there, or lie.

During any fertility cycle I felt like I was existing in a parallel universe. I physically participated in daily life, but I wasn't fully present in heart or mind. It was a peculiar distanced feeling. You do what you do to get through in the best way you can.

I was genuinely fearful that I would transform into a raging, hormonal monster and not cope on my own at the cottage for a week, so I asked Mum to come and stay with me. Bless her cotton socks, thankfully she agreed. I rang her that afternoon to announce we had the green light. I confirmed our accommodations, and booked my follicle tracking scans in Tamworth for the next Wednesday, Friday and following Monday, just so I was in their schedule. I was in my element – making plans. That night I savoured my last delicious glass of wine and it tasted like the end of a chapter.

The next few days passed in a blur of packing, cleaning and organising preparing to leave for Bendemeer. I had been loving the rigorous exercise and meal plan I'd been following, but it was back to the maintenance nutrition plan and walking only now. Overall, I was feeling good, though perhaps a bit hyped with anticipation and the chasm of unknown ahead of me. I was also a bit emotional, crying at ads on TV, but that wasn't terribly unusual for me.

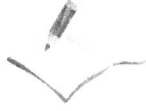

17/06/13 CYCLE DAY 5 (DAY 4 of FSH) Monday

- *Blood test this morning*
- *Starting to get lots of pimples on my face*
- *Feeling normal, maybe a little bit PMT-ish with a short temper and emotional*
- *Mum & I drove to Bendemeer to stay at the cottage for this week. We arrived later than expected – 5:45pm after a 4.5hr drive – about an hour longer than expected.*
- *Before leaving I had some work to do, got my car rego sorted, Ad and I spoke to our Accountant re: pre-EOFY tax planning, had blood test, got a few more groceries, then had lunch and finished packing. Busy day!*
- *Received word that I have been accepted to speak on branding at the Pharmacy Business Network Conference in Canberra in September – very excited! I was invited last week and submitted a proposal.*
- *Had a call from Genea saying they received our consent & agreement forms (which we'd signed) but the signatures weren't witnessed so we need to sign them again and scan and email by the end of the week, then take originals with us to Sydney...grrrr! We might have to head back to Goondi on Friday because of that.*
- *Ad in Moree for work. I didn't get to say goodbye to him this morning before he left (I was down the street) and felt very sad. I feel like at the moment I don't want to be apart from him. He's in Moree for 2 nights, then back to Goondi on Wednesday.*
- *I'm glad Mum is here. We had dinner with the owners of the farm and cottage tonight. It is freezing cold… -4 degrees here so we've got electric blankets and heaters on flat out!*

18/06/13 CYCLE DAY 6 (DAY 5 of FSH) Tuesday

- *Had an easy day at the cottage doing some work. Did my first business coaching call with a client today. Ended up being a productive work day, luckily we have phone and internet reception. Mum relaxed, reading and doing patchwork.*

- *Results of yesterday's blood test showed my oestrogen = 350. Next BT and first scan on Friday morning. Sunday could be the soonest we go to Sydney but we won't know for sure until Friday. We'll head back to Goondi on Friday to get papers signed, then I'll return on Sunday.*

- *Feeling good, few crampy feelings in lower back and right ovary. Start Orgalutran needles in the morning.*

. . .

I celebrated my 32nd birthday on the chilly winter's day labelled in my journal as Cycle Day 7 (Day 6 of FSH). I still didn't have a baby and the clock was still ticking, but guess what… the world hadn't ended.

I administered my first Orgalutran® injection that morning which left a red mark around the site and a peppery taste in my mouth (happy birthday to me!). The needle hurt more than Puregon so I wasn't much of a fan of it! It even sounds like a wicked name, like Orgalutran should be the name of a new decepticon Transformer®. It's an antagonist to prevent ovulation before the desired time. It was laughable that I was jabbing myself to avoid ovulating when for years that's all I wanted.

It was a hectic birthday spent like this: a coaching teleclass at 7am I dialled in for wrapped in blankets, breakfast, needles, birthday present opening, then to Tamworth for acupuncture at 10am, shopping, lunch with Mum and two of my closest friends, appointment with Rhonda from Genea to pick up more drugs, a short catch up with a family friend, more shopping and home at 5:45pm. The only thing missing was seeing my darling. It was strange to have a birthday without him.

I felt generally unwell that evening which was due to one or more of the following: the Orgalutran, overdoing it that day, being tired, slightly overwhelmed, dehydrated and emotional. Possibly a combination of all of them. Some cramping in my lower back had started and with each cramp the reality of IVF became more real. I was doing a lot of speculating about the week ahead, countered with "One day at a time Benita, one day at a time."

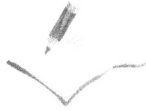

20/06/13 CYCLE DAY 8 (DAY 7 FSH) Thursday

- *Uneventful day here at the cottage. We slept in, had a late breaky, then I worked for the day while Mum read, did patchwork and relaxed. I went for a walk this afternoon and we semi-packed the car to leave in the morning.*
- *Few small twinges and cramps today, but feeling good otherwise. Praying I have a nice batch of follicles developing that we'll see on the ultrasound scan in the morning.*
- *Leaving some gear here since we'll be back on Sunday.*

. . .

Cycle Day 9 (Day 8 FSH) was follicle tracking scan day and my anxiety was sky high. What if I didn't have any follicles? What if they weren't growing? What if I had too many? What was it all going to mean?

We got the early morning blood test out of the way before my scan. As accustomed as I was to having these scans, I never reached the point of being totally comfortable with nakedness from the waist down in a room with a stranger. Then there was that awkward moment when the sonographer would ask, "Would you like to insert the probe or should I?" My response was always, "You do it please." I had become a master at small talk and sarcastic remarks to make everyone (or maybe just me) feel better and fill the nervous gap between the beginning and the outcome.

Follicles contain follicular fluid and are seen as tiny black bubbles via ultrasound. I watched in amazement as they appeared on the screen set up for patient viewing. We saw some black bubbles on the left ovary and some black bubbles on the right. You little beauty! The sonographer counted 12 follicles of a reasonable size in total.

Mum and I had a five hour trip back to Goondiwindi Friday afternoon, and by the time we arrived I was tired, cranky and feeling yukky. It was so great to see Ad, though he was stressed with end of financial year responsibilities and worked until late that night. It seemed to me that he was not thinking about IVF at all and it was business as usual for him.

I received a call from Genea en route to say they had my result from that morning (that was fast) and I would need a blood test Sunday morning. They suggested it might be best to head to Sydney on Sunday in readiness for the BT and scan following that. Crikey, now I had to find accommodation in Sydney fast. I hadn't booked anything yet because how do you make a booking when you don't know when you'll arrive or how long you'll be there, or even if the accommodation will be needed at all if the cycle fails? I spent a few hours that evening trying to find an apartment in Sydney that was available, of reasonable quality and price, self-contained and had parking and proximity to public transport. I was fairly clueless about Sydney so it was a challenge.

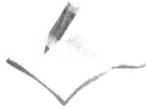

22/06/13 CYCLE DAY 10 (DAY 9 FSH) Saturday

- *Up and pretty much straight into continuing the search for Sydney apartment. Took me hours! Still in PJ's at 12:30 when dropped Ad to rugby and still hadn't started packing. Agghhh…was very stressed! Ad played rugby while I eventually got apartment in Elizabeth Bay booked, had a shower, dressed, ate, and started to get gear packed, while trying to get 4 loads of washing dry. Ad's team won footy vs Condamine (playing 2nd grade today) and we left home at 4pm. Had a good trip to Bendemeer, watched British Lions game vs Wallabies (we lost 23-21) at the Bendemeer pub and had a delicious lamb roast meal! Got out to the cottage at 10pm and were in bed by 10:45pm.*

- *Very teary (crying over everything) + feeling bloated and crampy*

. . .

Cycle Day 11 (Day 10 FSH) was drive to Sydney day. After the final freezing night at the farm cottage, we were off and racing to my 8:30am blood test in Tamworth and a takeaway coffee pitstop. Heading to Sydney meant it was all really happening. I wondered how many times we would have to do this, and how many times we could afford to. We were pleasantly surprised that with Australia's Medicare rebate, and our private health insurance, IVF was not as costly as we first thought. My uneducated assumption was that it would cost about $10,000 per round, but it was more like half that, so that was a huge relief. Even so, it was money we had to find.

During our drive I had a somewhat diplomatic chat to Ad about showing more compassion toward me. He had been preoccupied with work and we'd been apart a lot in the past month, so I felt he'd not really acknowledged what I was going through. I wondered if it was callous of me as I knew that it was a difficult time for him too and how could he know what it felt like when he wasn't experiencing the physical side of it like I was? I am the only one in my body to feel the way I felt. I was the only one who could produce eggs and carry our baby. There was no escaping the fact that in many regards I had to go through it alone. Had I been communicating with him effectively? Perhaps he could have tried harder to understand? He took what I said to heart and it reminded me that we simply need to be straight up with the men in our lives as they are often not great at guessing games.

What I didn't see, because he didn't show it, and I was too blinded by my own self-absorption, was the toll IVF took on Adam. It just looked different. I saw him still working full time, still playing sport and going about his normal life. And truth be told I was a little bit resentful of that. What I didn't see was the strain on him to uphold his relatively new job without people knowing his private business. I didn't see the weight on his shoulders to keep money coming in to fund our treatments when I had cut back my Sunburnt Country work hours. And he was part of the process too, with the same hopes and disappointments I had.

The button on my jeans was undone the whole way to Sydney to accommodate my swollen tummy. We reached our apartment at about 3pm in the pouring rain to discover it was in a beautiful spot on the marina at Elizabeth Bay. However, there was no parking available anywhere for more than one hour without a permit. Aghhh… we were such rookies. After a bit of panicking, we worked out we could leave our car at my friend Mandy's house. She came and picked it up and saved our bacon. The apartment was nice, comfortable and quiet, but not properly cleaned (private AirBnB rental), so we vacuumed and cleaned the toilet (just what I felt like – as if we hadn't already had a big enough day).

Genea called with my blood test result and advised that the egg retrieval procedure would be on Tuesday morning. I was to have my ovulation trigger needle at 7:15pm that night and Ad had to ejaculate. My oestrogen level had doubled in the past 48 hours (that was good), but it didn't seem to be as high as other results I was reading online. I hoped that wasn't a bad sign. I allowed myself (and kind of stuck to) only 15 minutes per day perusing online IVF forums because it was a source of confusion and undue worry. I sought comfort in other women's comparable results so that it might be an indicator of an outcome for us. I came to realise this wasn't the case because it's such an individual experience with many variables.

I felt dizzy, bloated and sick to my stomach about 5:30pm, as was becoming the norm for that time of day. A shower, food and water helped after the commotion of the day.

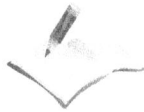

24/06/13 CYCLE DAY 12 (no needles) Monday

- *It was a challenge to walk up the hill to the coffee shop...I was totally breathless!*

- *Gee, it was good not to have any needles today after 4 of them yesterday. Really what have I got to complain about compared to people who are sick or have serious health concerns? Needles are no fun but not that bad really, either.*

- *Quiet day in our apartment both working on our laptops and phones. The beauty of technology, eh! We went out for a coffee, but that was the only time we left. Mandy and Brody came over and cooked us dinner – yummy steak and veg with a Dijon mustard type sauce. It was a team effort and a nice distraction.*

- *Feeling bloated and moody (poor Adam!) but otherwise okay.*

- *Our IVF egg retrieval is in the morning. Our first and hopefully only time. We need to be at Genea at 6:30am, so have booked a taxi to pick us up at 6:10am. I can't believe that after all the months of waiting, planning, wondering and worrying, and these last few weeks of needling,*

driving, tests and scans, the time has finally arrived. This is the
procedure I have been most scared about, until today. I don't know
how to describe it; it's like calm has washed over me. My resilience
and strength have surfaced, telling me I will get through this time no
matter what. Telling me that no matter what experience and outcome
we encounter, I am strong, I have a Davis and Bensch ticker and I will
be okay. I am not afraid of the pain – physical, mental or emotional
– I will endure and overcome. The prize at the end of this road will
be worth more than any pain I could go through. I feel selfish talking
about myself a lot and not including Adam much. He is such a part
of this and feeling the strain as well. He's also a great support to me.
I'd like to think we're a great support to each other. My strength comes
from within and that is what I draw on at times like this, more than
reaching out for anyone or anything. Dear Lord, please take care of us.

. . .

The twenty-fifth of June 2013 was Cycle Day 13 and egg retrieval day. The next step in the process. Another step closer to our baby. As much as we took the process into our hands, the unknown still remained. We could be days away from pregnancy or still months… years… When I woke at 2:45am to check the clock, I pleaded with myself not to get carried away with the 'what ifs' and focus on the present moment – go back to sleep!

My alarm sounded at 5:15am and I had that strange feeling you get sometimes when you don't know if you've been asleep or not. Anyway, time was of the essence so I showered, we had breakfast and got ready for the taxi to collect us at 6:10am. We'd allowed 20 minutes to get to Genea, but were there in five, so had 15 minutes to wait and let my nerves brew.

At 6:30 we used our access card to go up the lift onto the day surgery floor, and found our way into the right waiting room to fill out paperwork. From there, we were taken through to a tiny dressing room to put covers over our shoes, pants off (for me that is – I felt like I was continually taking my pants off for someone), gowns on and to place our belongings into a designated locker. We were led into the preparation/recovery area where we walked past other couples who were in their own curtained off spaces like the one we were going to. Some we could see through the cracks in the curtain, others we could only hear. The look in their eyes was mirrored in ours. I wondered who they were, where they'd come from, what was their story. Was this their first time like us? Had they been here ten times already? I wanted to reach out to every one of them and I hoped they could feel the silent love I was sending them. There's a good chance they thought I was just a bit creepy looking in at them.

After we got settled in our curtained space, we were paid a visit by Dr. Livingstone who explained what was going to happen. I just wanted to get it over and done with by this stage. We were in the theatre room by 7:15am. There were three people in there with us: Dr. Livingstone, a nurse and the lovely embryologist Sara. It was dimly lit and I felt like I was going in for an operation except for the fact that I entered the room in an upright position. Up onto the reclining seat I went with my feet in stirrups (they didn't tell me that part. Didn't they know I wasn't here to give birth? Bye dignity). I shut my eyes momentarily. "Think about something else Benita, think about something else."

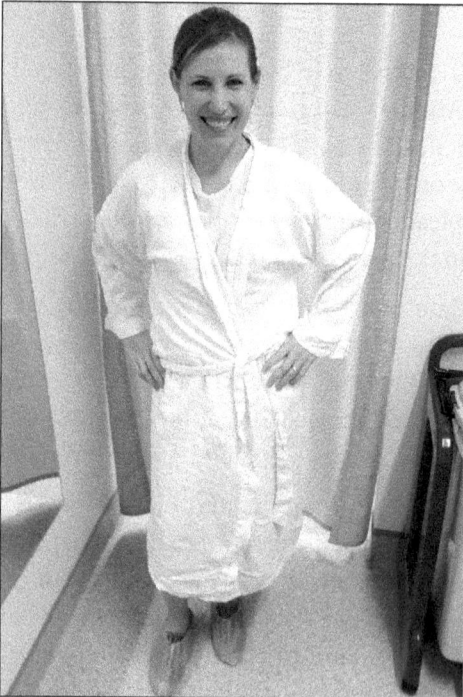

Looking more confident than I felt prior to my first egg retrieval at Genea, Sydney June 2013.

I was given a sedative through a canula in my hand, and at some point I had a local anaesthetic down below. I felt a little woozy but was still fully aware of what was happening and what I was saying. I remember smiling goofily, a lot. It was incredible to watch the ultrasound screen near my head and witness Dr. Livingstone extracting the fluid from my follicles one by one from each ovary. Then the nurse would pass the test tubes filled with follicle fluid to the embryologist, and she would look for eggs. I hoped the nurse had steady hands.

It was nowhere near as bad as I anticipated – over in 10 minutes and a far cry from the level of pain I had braced myself for. The most I felt was discomfort rather than distinct pain. Dr. Livingstone was quick, efficient and experienced, and he put me at ease. I had 12 follicles retrieved which resulted in 10 eggs (one of them potentially immature). We were delighted. Although one egg can be all that's needed for a successful IVF cycle, it's a bit of a numbers game whereby not all eggs go on to be fertilised or result in viable embryos, so starting with more is normally better.

After the procedure Dr. Livingstone pushed me in a wheelchair back into our curtained space and I was delivered tea and biscuits. Ad was taken away to give his 'sample' five minutes later. During his absence, the embryologist came to tell me we got 10 good quality eggs and some other info that started to blur together through a rush of nausea. She called a nurse who quickly tipped me back, gave me a shot of nausea medication and told me to take deep breaths. I was okay within a few minutes. Ad came back soon after, we got our recovery instructions, had a cuppa and yarn and left in a taxi at 8:50am.

Back at our apartment, we watched a movie and then I spent the afternoon in bed because the pain in my lower abdomen and back kicked in after the medication wore off. Panadol and heat packs were my friends. By dinner time I didn't need any more pain relief, so it wasn't too serious. The physical side of IVF was a nice distraction from the mental and emotional, as sometimes the head fuck was almost too much to bear. It was actually good to feel it in my body rather than only in my mind.

We received the news the next morning that eight of our eggs had fertilised naturally. We had no preconceived expectations, but 80% seemed fantastic. Go Ad's swimmers! We were thrilled, and particularly so that intracytoplasmic sperm injection (ICSI) hadn't been required. This day was classed as day 1 for our little embryos. We prayed that they were multiplying as they should in their little dishes in the incubator at Genea. I felt like I should be there with them. It was an extremely unusual feeling not to be and I felt a strong pull on my heart. I tried not to dwell on that part of it, that our potential future baby (or babies) was growing outside of me, without me, in a glass dish. I knew they were being taken good care of, but it wasn't by me. It just wasn't… natural. All we could do was wait for the call on Friday (day 3 for the embryos) to tell us how they were progressing.

I was bloated and sore so the day was spent working at my laptop, dotted with two breaks for a short walk and fresh air. Adam did the same and spent 80% of his day (talking loudly) on the phone. The busyness of our little apartment helped to keep our mind off the obvious. The upside of this experience was time spent with Adam in a pretty spot with access to takeaway food and coffee just down the road.

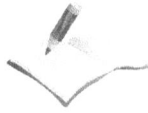

27/06/13 Day 2 for embryos

- *Bloated tummy (unchanged) and some mild cramping. Only able to walk slowly and short distances before I get short of breath and feel a bit yukky.*

- *We worked until 1:30pm and then headed into the city (via a train from Kings Cross Station). I'd never been to Kings Cross before…it is exactly as you think it is… my perception has been shaped from the Underbelly TV series. I had an acupuncture appt. at 2:30 and Ad had a massage for his tight calf, hamstring and back muscles. The acupuncture was great. We then watched 'Man of Steel' (the new Superman movie) at the cinema at 4:30, headed back to Kings Cross and had a delicious Japanese meal at a local restaurant here in Elizabeth Bay. Tomorrow we'll receive a call from the scientists updating us on our embryos' progress – how many are developing well, or not.*

- *Had 6 clicks of Ovidrel injection today to help with uterus lining developing at optimum for nourishing a baby*

28/06/13 Day 3 for embryos

- *A cool rainy day in Sydney. I didn't leave the apartment all day. Ad went for a run for 45 minutes at 5pm. Had a good work day, achieving what I needed to. We went out for tea in Randwick to a*

Spanish tapas bar with Mandy and Brody. It was so yummy. They took us out for gelato afterwards... also delicious. My tummy is so full and bloated, but now I can't tell if it's the dinner or the follicle fluid. It's bloody tight nonetheless. Getting some odd cramps in lower abdomen and back but nothing serious.

- *Feeling hormonal and moody today. Short fuse. Also a bit flat.*
- *Got our day 3 results from Genea:*
  - *8 embryos fertilised. 1 arrested = 7 remaining*
    - *2 embryos 6 cells in size*
    - *2 embryos 7 cells in size*
    - *1 embryo 8 cells in size*
    - *2 embryos 4 cells in size (too small, outside acceptable range, won't make it)*
- *Days 3-5 is the big step as they need to divide to about 100 cells at day 5 to be blastocysts. Praying we get one good, strong, viable blastocyst and if we could have one or more to freeze that would be amazing. We won't know until Sunday. Tomorrow we'll find out our transfer time for Sunday.*

. . .

The day before our embryo transfer I hit a wall, figuratively speaking. I was tired, emotional, moody and anxious with bloating and regular cramps. I had planned to visit an old Uni friend but cancelled, as I couldn't cope with being out and about with the hassle of city driving and parking. I stayed in to relax while Ad went to a college alumni function at Bondi. It was a smart decision.

Diverting my energy inward was exactly what I needed. I found a fabulous blog online at www.catchingrainbowsfertility.co.uk that helped me so much to get into a positive mind frame conducive to accepting our embryo. I also downloaded some Circle + Bloom guided meditations from www.circlebloom.com which I listened to and copied over to my phone. I finished my 'me' time feeling a lot better with a positive mindset and new tools to support me. This was my first exposure to pregnancy affirmations which I continued to embrace daily. I felt in control of my mind again and was ready for our embryo transfer. The online pregnancy due date calculator calculated that our baby would be due 18/03/14.

Sunday the thirtieth of June was day 5 for our embryos and the day the strongest would be transferred into my uterus. Was it the day my wish would come true? Was it so simple that after all the trying I could wander into the procedure un-pregnant and wander out pregnant? I worried for a long time that allowing myself to believe it would happen would mean a harder fall if it didn't. But if I didn't allow myself to believe, then it was more likely not to happen. I decided I had to expect the best. I had to expect this was the day. I had to put it all on the line and get my mind right to allow my body the best chance of receiving this baby.

I didn't sleep well the night before the transfer and we were early to pack our car, leave our apartment (in the rain again) and find parking near Genea. We were inside Genea at 8:10 ready for my pre-transfer acupuncture appointment at 8:30. I listened to a guided meditation during acupuncture which helped me to stay calm and hone my thoughts in on welcoming our embryo.

The trickiest part of an embryo transfer has nothing to do with the transfer itself – it's managing the full bladder situation. Our transfer was booked for 9:30am. I was meant to do a pee at 8:30 and then drink 500ml of water, but because of my acupuncture appointment I did a pee at 8:15 and drank half of it, then practically sculled the rest when I got out at 8:55. My bladder was meant to be full, but it was uncomfortably full. It was difficult to concentrate on anything else and I was so worried I wouldn't able to hold it. Dr. Livingstone said I "overachieved in the bladder stakes!"

The procedure only took about 10 minutes and was very similar to the IUI procedures I'd had in the past. No drugs involved, just a speculum and the blastocyst embryo inserted through the cervix and into the uterus. The embryologist came to talk to us beforehand and told us we had a grade 1 embryo to transfer (the one that was eight cells at day 3). They called it a "lovely embryo" so that sounded good to us. Must be going to be a girl! We had been given the choice of transferring more than one embryo, but we decided on what was recommended for us – one. Silent tears of joy slipped from the corners of my eyes as I watched the incredible spectacle of a new life being placed in his/her new home. Despite the obstacles of IVF and it not being our preferred method of achieving a baby, it was certainly a highlight to see my eggs during the egg retrieval and then our embryo during the embryo transfer. I was very grateful for modern medicine.

I pretty much bolted (well as quickly as I could shuffle in my gown) to the toilet immediately after the procedure although I was nervous about getting up straight away... would the embryo fall out? Dr. Livingstone assured me it wouldn't, and I wondered whether other crazy hormonal ladies asked him that.

After a cup of tea and receiving our instructions, it was back to acupuncture for me. This was a much more relaxing session than the pre-transfer one in which I'd felt so sensitive to the needles.

I read somewhere that I should keep my feet warm during and after the transfer. I had a special pair of red merino woollen socks from Maria that I kept on until we arrived in Goondiwindi at 8:30pm. Thankfully Adam was happy to drive the whole way while I slept, dozed, ate, chatted and gazed out the window. I was so relieved we'd done all the hard parts that we had control over and, my goodness, it was good to be home.

I told myself, "I have our baby in my uterus." Was it possible to already love this little ball of cells? To me it was.

**For detailed medical notes from this IVF cycle please see the Appendix.

A special note on trying not to headbutt someone

There are a lot of things people don't tell you about the challenging journey to conception. One of them is how you will sometimes have the inclination to yell at and/or headbutt someone. That someone may be your husband, friend, mother, the nearest pregnant person or even a complete random who just so happens to be in your line of sight. No matter how much you may want to lash out when the feeling takes you, you are customarily forced to suppress it.

I recall many instances of overwhelming, irrational rage stemming from some menial thing, or no good reason at all. One such instance was dropping in to get a few things from the local supermarket after a blood test during one treatment cycle. The supermarket was undergoing a revamp at the time and some of my usual items had been relocated. Ordinarily, when in my good-natured, unmedicated state (exception: PMT at its worst), this wouldn't bother me. However, on this day it took everything in my power not to unleash an almighty scream and throw a tantrum on the floor because I couldn't find what I was looking for. This is when I realised I needed to go straight to the checkout, walk directly to the car, load it and drive home.

The rage could also be triggered by questions and comments made with little or no thought, like, "When are you having a baby?" and "Come on, you better hurry up!"

I became more thick-skinned with time and could mostly handle these comments with a flippant, "Don't worry, we're trying," and a swift change of subject. On the inside my voice yelled, "You have no bloody idea what we're going through!"

I was shocked at how thoughtless people could be at times. It pained me to think of all the other women out there also dealing with this on a daily basis.

I came to be better at smiling and nodding when people would say things like, "It will happen when it's ready," or "Now that you're more relaxed it might just happen."

When I was in the right frame of mind, I'd let these remarks run off. When I was loaded with hormones, I struggled not to headbutt said person and scream at them, "Don't you think I've been relaxed at some point in the last two years?"

"Stay positive," was another classic. When someone said "stay positive" to me, through gritted teeth I would think, "I am trying to stay positive! You bloody try and stay positive all the time." This was up there as the most infuriating comment to swallow.

Although what I desired was to be and stay positive, I had to allow myself to feel negative sometimes. I had to give myself permission to feel whatever it was that I felt at that point in time. I couldn't beat myself up if I wasn't in a perpetual state of positivity. I taught myself to sit in the negativity sometimes and trust that I'd soon be back on the other side.

People are mostly good and mean well. I 100% understand that the abovementioned types of questions and comments are not meant to harm and that people generally don't know what to say. It's the best support they can muster with their level of awareness.

In regards to another individual's child-bearing status (none, one or more children), of any age, my view is this: **Unless information is offered to you by that individual, any questions you might wish to ask are better left unasked, and any comments you might wish to express are better left unsaid.** Exercise self-restraint.

P.S. No one was actually physically headbutted in the making of this story, in case you are wondering.

CHAPTER 9

Trying with IVF 2WW

The dreaded two week wait (which is actually less than two weeks in IVF cycles) began as soon as our microscopic embryo was deposited into its new home. I'd had more 2WWs than I cared to remember, but this was the BIG one. There were no more injections, scans or procedures to divert my attention, just almost two weeks with me and my mates: waiting, and Crinone®. Crinone is a progesterone gel I had to insert vaginally twice per day to help my uterus support a pregnancy. Its common side effects are cramps, headaches, feeling sad, unworthy (what!?) and emotional (great!), so that was something to look forward to (not).

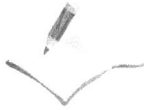

01/07/13 Day 1 Post Transfer

- *Slept in after 9 hours of much needed sleep and had an easy day at home working and doing a few jobs around the house*
- *Still bloated and experienced cramps in lower back and abdomen. Nothing severe, just a dull ache. Went to bed with a hot pack on my back.*
- *Very tired by the end of the day*
- *Started daily meditation and Crinone gel 90mg (8%) twice/day*

A few days in I decided to name it the 2 Week Date (with myself) instead of the 2 Week Wait. I set out to embrace the time to nourish my mind and body and give pregnancy the best chance possible. Fitting around my work, this was my 2 Week Date game plan:

- Go for nice gentle walks
- Meditate every day (using a Catching Rainbows rainbow meditation and the Circle + Bloom IVF mind + body program I'd downloaded)
- Eat delicious, nutritious food
- Sleep well
- Write in my journal
- Send positive energy, health, love and encouragement down to my uterus (non-trying people would think this is slightly nuts)

On day 2 post transfer I received a call from Genea embryology to inform us that one of our embryos, classed as grade 2, had been suitable for freezing and was 'placed on ice' on the day of our transfer. This was terrific news to have this embryo available for a frozen embryo transfer in the future. The embryologist went on to say that the blastocyst we'd had transferred had started to hatch when the transfer was performed, so should be implanting any time now. Oh my! Burrow in you little princess. I talked to her in my mind, telling her how much her Dad and I loved her, how special she was, and comforting her that my uterus was a wonderful place to settle in for nine months. I made the conscious decision to adopt the mindset that I was pregnant, so I practised thinking, speaking and journaling from that perspective. I was able to actually believe it probably 65% of the time. My self-mastery wasn't good enough to achieve 100%.

It was impossible to know whether my still bloated tummy and lower back/abdominal cramps were due to the progesterone or the aftermath of the procedures. Probably both, I thought. I felt a bit yuk that morning, just off and slightly nauseous. I hoped it was because our baby was implanting but as Ad said, "Don't read it into it too much." Fair point well made. It didn't stop me from spending 15 minutes on the internet researching 'feeling sick on implantation day' though. Ha.

The blood test at the IVF finish line was set for the eleventh of July. It couldn't come fast enough. Would I have the willpower to hold out and not do a pregnancy test at home before that? I hadn't made up my mind.

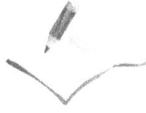

03/07/13 Day 3 Post Transfer

- *So tired tonight!*
- *Boobs started to hurt from time to time. Few mild cramps in the PM. Felt more energetic today and went for a walk down the street for lunch. Had 1hr sleep after meditating this morning, then did a webinar. This afternoon/tonight was working on planning and scheduling for July through till 8:30pm. Cooked a cake for Kylee's birthday tomorrow when she, Anthony and kids are here. Also had coaching reading to do. Ad away tonight. I am so ready for bed.*

. . .

Overnight between day 3 and day 4 post transfer I had vivid dreams, a few trips to the toilet and woke at 2:30am with stomach pain that continued for an hour before I drifted back to sleep. Of course, I was scrutinising every symptom – were these side effects of the Crinone, or pregnancy symptoms? The headfuck of trying with IVF continued. I started to question if the bloating was ever going away. It was okay in the morning but worsened as the day went on. I was also experiencing cramps, shortness of breath, a racing heart and needing to pee a lot. I was thinking about our baby a lot and wondering what was going on in there…

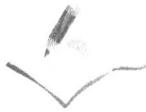

05/07/13 Day 5 Post Transfer

- *Feeling yukky today – dull pain in the tummy that lasted all day, like mild nausea*
- *Cramps in lower back and abdomen off and on and generally feeling lethargic*

- *Did not achieve much workwise before lunch, but got into it between 12 and 6pm and felt better in the afternoon, but then worse again at night*
- *Watched a movie in the night and took it easy*
- *On the countdown to pregnancy blood test, but actually not dwelling or stressing about it. I know I'm pregnant and it's easy to stay distracted.*

. . .

The sixth of July started very normally but wouldn't end that way. It was meant to be a typical Saturday rugby game day in Toowoomba that followed the standard format: drive to rugby ground, watch Adam play rugby and drive home.

On the two-and-a-half hour drive to Toowoomba I noticed how exceptionally bloated my tummy was. After days of wondering if it should still be like that I said to Ad, "I think I better call and check that this is normal." I rang Genea at 11am and described what I was experiencing. The nurse I spoke to was quick to conclude I had symptoms of ovarian hyper stimulation (OHSS). What the!? She requested I have a blood test that day to check my blood wasn't dehydrated, because the swelling in my abdomen was due to fluid being taken from my blood. Oh terrific, another blood test. It was a stroke of luck that we were in Toowoomba, so I had access to more collection centres. However, they all closed at noon and I wouldn't make it by then, so I dropped Adam at rugby and it was off to the Emergency department at the Toowoomba Hospital for me.

At 2:30pm I was still waiting for the blood test which would quantify my oestradiol, progesterone, haematocrit (HCT), and hCG levels. hCG – whoa, whoa, whoa… that's not for another five days, that's not part of the process. I was not ready to deal with that yet but it seemed I had no choice but to face it then and there.

While I waited, I Googled OHSS and read as much as I could on the topic. I self-diagnosed myself as having a mild case of OHSS, which… (drum roll please)… can be a positive indicator of pregnancy (!!!). Pregnancy kick starts OHSS 4-6 days after an embryo transfer due to hCG production. The downside was that increased hCG production leads to worse OHSS so this wasn't going to go away if I was pregnant. And there can be complications with OHSS so it was to be taken seriously. The first most critical immediate factor was ascertaining how hydrated my blood was. They drew a vial of blood and I continued my wait.

Adam was catching a lift to the hospital after rugby at the same time the doctor called me to discuss the blood test result. I swallowed hard. The blood work concluded I was not dehydrated so that was good. He then said, very matter-of-factly, like he was updating me on the football score, "Your bhCG is 31 today." It sounded like he assumed I knew this already. Did I hear him correctly?

"Does that mean I'm pregnant?"

"That is in line with very early pregnancy levels," he said while busily doing something else. He was not at all interested in involving himself in the emotions of it, so I kept mine in check too. He gave me the computer printout which I clutched tightly in my sweaty hand.

Well there you go, I thought. That was NOT how I was expecting to find out if IVF had worked for us: on my own in Toowoomba Hospital Emergency face-to-face with a random doctor! No build up, no mind games, BAM it was done. Ad arrived 10 minutes after I found out and was still in a daze. We walked outside past reception and I pulled out the printout to explain it to him. He looked at me quizzically "so that means…?" I nodded. We exchanged a big Adam Bensch bear hug. He was not expecting this news today either! According to one website I was only 3 weeks 4 days pregnant so it was very early days. It's a positive and a negative with IVF that you find out you're pregnant so early on. Positive in that you're dying to know, and negative in that it makes for a very long pregnancy.

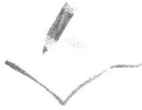

07/07/13 Day 7 Post Transfer

- *Rest day at home. Rested apart from folding clothes, washing up and cooking pumpkin soup. Drank 2250mL water.*

- *Dr. Liv rang to explain OHSS condition and let me know about early positive pregnancy result. These were the key points:*

  – *OHSS for me was due to pregnancy not hormone levels during IVF*

  – *Will be a "rough week"*

– Blood test in morning to check HCT and hCG

– If my blood becomes dehydrated, I'll be hospitalised

– Maximum rest but not total bed rest as don't want blood clots developing

– Start on daily Clexane injection, which is a blood thinner, to prevent clots. Had to go to Goondi hospital to get it as no pharmacies open today.

– Still experiencing abdo swelling, mild pains in lower abdo + back, mild nausea off and on. Uncomfortable to move around too much. I definitely feel better when reclined on the lounge. Some shortness of breath.

. . .

My ovaries hurt so much the day after the hospital adventure. I was terrified I was going to twist one or rupture a cyst or something else that I'd been reading about to do with mild-moderate OHSS that sounded horrid and painful. It wasn't much fun, but if it meant I was pregnant, then it was worth it. IVF had been a continual process of ticking the boxes as we completed each stage and this felt like another box had been ticked. I had a good feeling about the pregnancy but didn't want to truly believe it until I'd had a few more blood tests – one of which had been that morning. Waiting 24 hours for the result felt like an eternity.

Dr. Livingstone explained that late onset of OHSS is due to pregnancy and that it tends to get worse until the time of the pregnancy test, then will plateau and improve. Essentially what was happening was that my ovaries were enlarged, I had elevated hormone levels and the blood vessels in my ovaries were losing fluid into my abdomen. As a result, I needed to drink at least 2L of water a day and rest. The worst part about it was my abnormally large tummy – I looked about four months pregnant and if I did too much it was quite painful. I felt best reclined on the lounge which is what I was supposed to be doing. "Don't even do housework," the staff at Genea told me. It was the first time I experienced the addictive satisfaction of engaging a cleaner.

I cried six times that day. Some of it was unbridled hormones, some of it was worry and some of it was feeling downright rotten. I was so scared of something happening to endanger our baby. Keeping her was the most important thing in my world and I prayed for all to go well. I had my fingers crossed for the blood test result the following day and meanwhile had to front up again to inject my second daily Clexane® blood thinner injection.

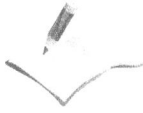

09/07/13 Day 9 Post Transfer (3w5d pregnant!)

- *Almost four weeks pregnant today (I think)! Only 36 weeks to go! Ha ha*

- *Had a better day today both emotionally and physically. Got blood test results from Monday (8th): HCT = normal, hCG = 66, Prog + oestrogen normal*

- *So, the great news is that our little bub's hCG more than doubled in the last 48 hours. I actually calculated the doubling rate to be 38 hours. This is great as hCG should double every 48-72 hours to indicate healthy growth and development.*

- *Bloating the same, still mild pain and today had some dizziness and nausea in the arvo. Also, some sharp ovary pains off and on. Boobs are fuller and more veiny and hurt from time to time.*

- *Still on Crinone gel, Clexane injection daily (blood thinner), rest and drinking lots of H20*

- *Still working but taking it very easy.*

11/07/13

Ouch! My boobs are HURTING. I have had sensations in my breasts around the time of my period before, but they have never full blown hurt! Maybe this is a sign of things to come. If it means being pregnant and having our beautiful baby I'm not complaining.

I have spent hours tonight googling 'late onset OHSS,' 'late onset OHSS and pregnancy,' 'late onset OHSS and twins' searching for... I don't know what. Reassurance, more information, more hope? Tomorrow we will get the results of our #3 bhCG level and my HCT. The way I'm feeling today, I'm pretty sure our little jelly bean is a healthy viable pregnancy!

I assume my hCG levels are rising because I'm feeling worse today, not better. Mostly it's the pains in my stomach and ovaries that have been more intense and frequent today. I've also had some cramping in my lower back which always fills my heart with dread because that's the feeling I got before my miscarriage (and my period every month). My stomach is still uncomfortably tight and I feel best when I'm not moving around much. Thank goodness I can work from home. I really don't know how anyone could go to a workplace and work feeling like this. I suppose women do it all the world over. There is nothing for it now but to give thanks, stay strong and positive and listen to my intuition. Everything is going to be just fine.

. . .

We truly could not believe how fortunate we were to become pregnant on our first IVF attempt. It was unexpected. We expected many more rounds. IVF is next level but our previous OI/IUI cycles certainly helped to prepare us for the all-consuming rigours of a stimulated cycle, for which I was grateful.

The OHSS eventually subsided, though I had prominent bloating for a few months. There came a time when the symptoms of OHSS and pregnancy blurred together and I didn't know which was causing what. For anyone with OHSS make sure you do as instructed, namely take it (really) easy and drink a lot of water. Also trust that things are going to get better really soon.

———

Post-OHSS I had a beautiful uncomplicated pregnancy until just before 36 weeks when things went a little pear shaped with sudden onset of pre-eclampsia and cholestasis of pregnancy.

I went into spontaneous labour and our precious son (my hunch was wrong) Bruce arrived pre-term on the twenty-first of February 2014 at 36 weeks and one day. He was big, strong and healthy with brown eyes and a full head of thick, black hair. Bruce established who was boss early on by firing his first pee at the paediatrician examining him. Every day since we have admired his thirst for knowledge, tenacity and beautiful big heart.

They say not to count your chickens before they hatch and it wasn't until our little chicken Bruce was hatched and in my arms that I truly allowed myself to believe we had done it. We had created a baby. I now had a place to belong; I could take my rightful place in the baby club.

Almost to the day it was 40 months since I threw the pill in the bin.

A special note to women in pain

For the beautiful women whose dreams have not come true…

I'm sorry that this happened for me and not for you.

I'm sorry for the suffering that you have endured.

I'm sorry for your loss.

I'm sorry that you grieve.

I'm sorry for the emptiness you feel.

I'm sorry that I don't have the answers.

I'm sorry I was not there for you in your time of need.

I'm sorry you did not get what you want.

I'm sorry I cannot take away your pain.

I'm so deeply sorry.

CHAPTER 10

Trying when the stakes aren't as high

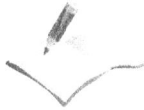

10/05/15

Today is Mother's Day 2015. Today my heart feels full and my eyes watery. I am feeling so much. I feel joy beyond comprehension when I look at our son, Bruce and feel him wriggling in my arms. I feel a love so full that it threatens to burst out of me. I feel gratitude so rich that it almost hurts. I thank God for the blessing of a healthy, happy little boy who, when he arrived almost 15 months ago, changed our world in an instant. I feel a deep sense of loss for the baby we lost; a yearning for him that will always remain. I feel a connection to the baby waiting for us on ice in Sydney; I feel her waiting for us to come back. I feel a craving for another baby. I feel the universe bringing her closer to us, yet she is asking me to play the waiting game again. The torturous confusing game that it is.

Here comes that word 'trying.' I am 'trying' to not let my thoughts run away from me. I am trying not to consider the 'what ifs' and not to hear the cascade of thoughts that are limiting. Instead I am trying to breathe and to believe that 'what will be, will be, in its own time.'

Trying for another baby is different than trying for the first. The definition of the worst case scenario changes: no longer is worst case being devastatingly childless, it is being the parents of an only child. And that's still a beautiful scenario.

The stakes aren't as high as they used to be once you've had a baby, but it doesn't change the deep longing for another child. I wanted four children. Adam wanted three, but after our track record, we agreed we'd take it one at a time and see how things went.

I secretly wanted to be pregnant by the time Bruce was six months old. I would daydream about unknowingly getting pregnant now that in my imagination I was a super-fertile-baby-producing-machine (even though I was still breastfeeding around the clock). I imagined myself, as I propped baby Bruce on one hip, slipping into conversations (with the flip of my hair) "oh yes, I got pregnant when Bruce was only three months old." Not that I physically wanted to be pregnant at that point, but what if I could be one of *those* incredible women who has two babies in a twelve month period. Could that be me now that we'd had our turn at infertility?

Other women would tell me "don't rely on breastfeeding as contraception, I got pregnant when I was breastfeeding…" And I'd think, "Awesome, bring it on!" Gosh, how I wanted to wear that achievement like a badge.

If I had any say in the matter, my preference was to have our second little person by the time Bruce was two. I wanted our children to be close-ish in age and I wasn't getting any younger so time was of the essence. The tarot card reader's prophecy was that we would have twins or two babies close together, so that lingered in the back of my mind. For many months I was convinced the Universe had things all sorted and 'proper trying' may not be necessary. We could wing it for a while.

We had a head start since this time around we knew it was at least possible for me to maintain a pregnancy and bring a healthy baby into this world. That was a huge comfort. We knew we *could* do it – with time, and maybe with help, but hopefully without. We also knew that we had a precious little Bensch embryo at Genea should we wish to use it, and that was a comfort too.

I felt a blissful absence of pressure when Bruce was a little baby and I still supposed that I would get pregnant effortlessly and accidentally. I trusted that it could happen for us… that it would happen.

But… then it didn't. I told myself "at least we have one." And I convinced myself of that.

Time went on and we still hadn't conceived. My trust in the magic of the Universe and my self-convincing argument that one is enough, both began to wane.

People would ask, "When are you going to have another one?" and I'd think, "Oh I'm planning on putting my order in online this weekend, so yeah about nine months from now. For fuck's sake I don't know when we're going to have another one people – it doesn't seem to be that simple!" Out loud I would laugh and brush the question off with something like, "Oh, we'll see."

As the months wore on my period returned, there was less breastfeeding, and the little trying voice starting saying, "Hellloooooooo I'm back…." I wanted to swat it away like a buzzing mosquito on a Queensland summer's night.

We hadn't used any contraception since his birth, but when Bruce was 10 months old we upped the ante and began trying a lot (i.e. timed intercourse). We were back to the ovulation guessing game (let's be honest – I hadn't missed that) and the mechanical sex, which was even more mechanical as I struggled to accept my new post-baby bits, all the new Mum feelings and body image issues. I didn't know exactly when, but I was fairly confident I was ovulating, because my period had become pretty regular since it returned eight months after Bruce's arrival.

It's a delicate topic the desire and ache for another baby whilst not wanting to appear ungrateful for the one you already have. You can't express to just anyone your unhappiness about it taking too long, because you encounter the reaction, "Oh well, at least you have one." I was acutely aware that some people don't even get one. That had been us at one point. So there was a huge ball of emotions involved, including guilt. I'd think, "I am grateful beyond belief for having Bruce, but that doesn't diminish my wanting a sibling for him."

My maternal instinct to procreate was very strong and when you really feel it, the number of children you already have doesn't seem to reduce it. Since having Bruce, I'd been convinced we'd conceive our second child naturally. I wanted so badly for that to be the truth and I believed that we could. We'd done it before. But the question was: did we want to wait?

What would it take to create our next little Bensch?

How long would it take?

Would we be patient and wait until it happened naturally?

What if it didn't?

Should we intervene and pay a visit to our dear Dr. Livingstone again?

Did we want to go down that path again?

Could we afford to?

These questions swirled around relentlessly. It began to get to me and once Bruce turned one, I could feel myself slipping ever so slightly down the treacherous slope of the black hole. Once again, I had set my expectations too high and was being forced to learn another lesson.

Tick, tick, tick.

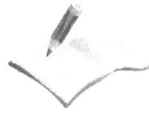

10/05/15 cont...

I had a pelvic ultrasound scan on day 14 last month and saw a lovely dominant 15mm follicle which is a good sign that I'm ovulating. All of that said, I don't know exactly WHEN I ovulate which has forever been my headache. We were having sex every day for a 4 or 5 day block around the middle of the month, but on advice from Dr. Livingstone last month went back to sex every 2nd day from approx days 10-18. Still no luck so far. I thought we may have succeeded this month, as, after 3 months of regular 29 day cycles, my period was late – 5 days late! There was no sign of it and I was having mild cramping in my lower back that would come and go (this accompanies my period, but I also had it in early pregnancy with Bruce). I did 3 preg tests that were all negative, so the wait was doing my head in and there was a glimmer of hope that maybe it was too early to test yet. I started to have some spotting and then yesterday my hopes were dashed. Sigh. Back to the start again, though it's a huge relief just to know so I can deal with it either way! I felt like a lunatic with raging hormones and a racing head for a few days, so it's a welcome release to hit the reset button on another month.

The little voice inside me suggested we keep trying naturally for a while longer, but the louder voice said, "get in and make it happen." Bruce was 14 months old, I was almost 34, and we wanted to get on with things. Who knew how long it was going to take to conceive again.

We were in the process of buying a farm near Moonie 130 kilometres northwest of Goondiwindi and were due to move there in late June. We'd be living an hour and 20 minute drive from town which made the logistics of a stimulated IVF cycle exponentially more stressful and complex. So, we made the decision and pulled the trigger on doing the cycle in June just before we started living permanently at the farm. Our plan was to pack and move all our gear to the farm before IVF, then during the IVF cycle stay with my little sister in Goondiwindi and then onto Sydney.

We had two options:

1) Do an unstimulated frozen embryo transfer and use the embryo we had on ice at Genea (easier, less risks and cheaper)
2) Do a stimulated IVF cycle, including an egg retrieval and embryo transfer like the last time

We chose the latter option to take the harder path first and hopefully the easier path later. My egg quality and quantity were diminishing every year, so it made sense to retrieve and store more at a younger biological age in case we needed them later. As soon as the decision was made, I started the wheels in motion organising the next few months.

Looking ahead I was not as overwhelmed by the process of IVF the second time around, but I *was* more apprehensive about the drugs and their effect on my body. It took its toll on me last time, exacerbated by OHSS – which I would likely experience again. But it was all worth it to grow our family.

Here we go again – more trying!

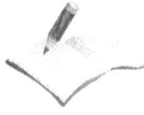

06/06/15

My period is due tomorrow and it will be day 1 of our IVF cycle. Yesterday we moved house. Today is like an in-between day – between the past and the future – as it always is, I guess!

CHAPTER 11

Trying with IVF the second time around

On Cycle Day 1, the seventh of June 2015, I drove 650km from Goondiwindi to Tamworth and back, to have my Day 1 blood test and pick up my IVF drugs from the Genea Tamworth office. I arrived home at 5pm exhausted and glad to cuddle Ad and my little Bruce man. I was also relieved that we were underway: my period had arrived, we knew the cycle was going ahead, and we could now make our plans.

IVF had snuck up on us since we'd been focused on the huge changes going on in our lives in the six weeks prior. Namely: the settlement of our new farm, starting to farm it around Adam's full time job, setting up the farming business, Adam preparing to finish his job, packing up our rental house in Goondiwindi, and moving our belongings to the farm. I was also working part time in Sunburnt Country and Bruce was keeping me occupied for the remainder. It had been hectic to say the least, and before Day 1 I hadn't thought too much about what it actually meant to immerse myself in IVF again.

IVF the second time around felt different. It felt quite surreal, like another facet of my life to manage, not the centre of my life as it was the first time. It was no less important to us, no less unpredictable or gut-wrenching, but understanding the process counted for a lot. It's like baking a cake from a recipe you've used before. You're not totally sure what the cake will look and taste like, but the ingredients and method are familiar and you have the benefit of experience. I speculated about how it might feel when faced with the fifth or fifteenth round of IVF.

The daily FSH injections started, this time branded Gonal-F®, and I got underway with my daily guided meditations. I also started to refocus on my physical well-being as I'd let that slide in the franticness of recent events. We had temporarily moved in with my little sister Terri in her three bedroom house in Goondiwindi and basically taken it over with a destructive toddler. She was incredibly generous and patient allowing us into her space, helping with Bruce and also helping me to pack at our rental. I loved having Terri's company while Ad was away so much. It wasn't hard to abstain from intercourse (as instructed during IVF) when Ad was hardly around.

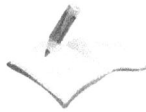

11/06/15 CYCLE DAY 5 (Day 4 of Gonal-F)

I had my Day 5 blood test today here in Gundy so that we can be sure Genea will receive the result tomorrow. Doing IVF in the bush really is a challenge...all the logistics are tricky! I've spent a considerable amount of time the past few days arranging to have my Day 8 and Day 10 scans and bloods in Moree (much closer than Tamworth), with my blood having to be collected there and transported to Tamworth for testing. After numerous calls, it turns out it won't work out with the couriers – either they don't run that day, won't deliver till that night or the next morning, or won't transport blood! Aggghhh – frustrating!

So, the new plan is to go to Tamworth after all! We'll drive down and back on Monday (tonight is Thursday) and then back again on Wednesday, hopefully stay with friends that night, then onto Sydney on Thursday. Need to start looking for a place to stay!

Generally feeling okay, but am getting occasional headaches, hot flashes and this morning some nausea, though that could have been due to having my needle before breakfast.

Lots of work on at the moment.

Early on in the cycle I sought shelter in the process, as I had in the past. I was in full-blown operational mode engrossed in the what, how and when of life. There was a lot to organise and do before we left Goondiwindi for Sydney. All I could see for the next fortnight was the strain of final packing, cleaning, moving, travelling and procedures, plus the physical effect of IVF and looking after Bruce through all of it. I felt tired in mind, body and spirit just thinking about it. I was really enjoying my Sunburnt Country work which, at the time, included a growing coaching clientele and a couple of interesting branding and communications projects. I probably didn't need the stress of deadlines at that time though. Adam was also under a lot of pressure in his sales manager role and getting things ticking over at the farm. Fortunately, we both had flexibility in our work and could work from anywhere providing we had our phones and computers. We pushed on as best we could and started to cross off the to-dos as we got further into the cycle, which gave us a feeling that things were slowly falling into place.

The IVF process was the same as our first round in 2013, except that this time I was liaising with Rhonda, the Genea nurse in Tamworth rather than the nurses at Genea Sydney. It was more personal and localised as Rhonda facilitated and supported other women from the area through fertility treatment every day of the week. I liked that I could visit her in person at the Tamworth office.

My early oestrogen level was discouraging and that made me very nervous. I tried to stay positive and prayed I had some beautiful little follicles growing. We'd soon see.

Adam, Bruce and I did another day trip to Tamworth on Day 8 for my blood test and first scan. The sonographer measured five follicles equal to and larger than 10mm (one on left ovary, four on right ovary). When Rhonda rang to discuss my results, she said they were "reasonable… maybe a bit on the low side." My heart sank. What did that mean? It wasn't disastrous, but it meant we may not have a lot of eggs to choose from and the cycle could be slower than expected (i.e. longer until the egg retrieval than we thought). I felt disheartened but as always, my voice of reason (Adam) kept things in perspective – "don't get ahead of yourself Benita, all we need is one good egg, so just wait and see." I was glad that I had *any* follicles but I'd be lying if I said I didn't want more.

There are some givens with every fertility treatment regardless of how busy you are and how many times you've been through it.

1) At some point all the emotions will kick in

2) At some point the plethora of physical side effects kick in too

As we got closer to the middle of the cycle, my emotions did start to kick in. There was a lot to handle at the time and the sentiment involved hit home: this wasn't just about booking appointments and driving here and there like a madwoman, we were trying to create a new life. Another child. And I had to face facts again that it may or may not work – this time, next time, or the one after that.

Perhaps I was simply a bit tired and overwhelmed, but as the days went on I started to feel like no one understood what it was like to go through this. People expected me to keep going along as per normal when I wanted them to acknowledge that it wasn't easy. Or was it my *own* expectation of myself to keep going along as per normal? Did I appear so capable and because we'd done it before that people thought "she'll be right mate." I was looking for more support from someone, but who? I wasn't good at directly asking for it, which was likely the problem.

It was a reality check when I started to feel in my body from Day 7 onwards the effect of the drugs and growing follicles. I thought, knowingly, "Oh goodness, that's right, I remember now what this feels like." From there the anticipation started to build.

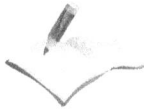

16/06/15 CYCLE DAY 10 (day 9 of Gonal-F)

It's all a bit much at the moment, but day by day and I just need to stay calm and focused on the outcome. Focused on why we're doing this and not just all the steps. Hoping that my oestrogen levels continue to go up and these little beautiful follicles are 5 perfect eggs. That would be wonderful. I did get a little bit emotional in the scan yesterday looking up on the screen, seeing my babies. I want to look after them the best way I can and hoping that they're growing beautifully as they should.

Our perfect little potential bubbas! Okay, I'll sign off for now and talk again soon.

. . .

On the seventeenth of June we travelled to Tamworth again for my Day 10 blood test and scan. The scan revealed nine follicles over 10mm including a dominant one measuring 19.7mm, so that was promising! We stayed with friends in Gunnedah for two nights before the next leg of the trip to Sydney. We wanted to stay away from the city rat race, and reduce our expenditure, as long as we could. On my 34th birthday (Day 12) we hit the road to Sydney via another blood test and scan early that morning in Tamworth. Here's an interesting fact I learned: the process of taking blood from a vein is called phlebotomy. I was very much feeling like a phlebotomist's pin cushion by this stage, with small bruises in the crevices of both my elbows.

I was to give myself the full pen of Ovidrel (the ovulation trigger injection) at 7:30pm on Saturday the twentieth, which was the second night we spent with our friends, Mandy and Brody, in Sydney. We checked into a very nice Waterloo apartment on Sunday for six nights to give ourselves a day to get sorted before the 7am Tuesday egg retrieval.

I couldn't believe how bloated my tummy was – I really did look pregnant! I felt very similar to how I did at the same point in our previous IVF round: tired, crampy, breathless and nauseous at times. I was keen to get the retrieval over and done with and was praying we had a good outcome. Ultimately all we needed was one good egg to transfer!

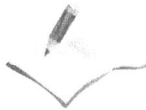

22/06/15 Cycle Day 15 Egg Retrieval Day

- *Bruce was looked after by Mandy. She arrived at 6:30am.*
- *Egg retrieval was at 7:30am this morning. 8 eggs were retrieved – Five that were really good and 3 that need to "catch up."*
- *Procedure itself was okay – spent more time on RHS ovary, only 2*

follicles on the LHS. Must be a longer, more painful procedure for women with 20-30 follicles.

- *Recovery is worse than the procedure, with nausea and pain in ovaries. We left Genea at 9:40, I had Panadeine Forte at Genea, 2x Panadiene at 12 noon, then have had 2 lots of Panadol this arvo/tonight.*
- *Now (11pm) feeling very bloated, but pain is mild*
- *Fertilisation results in morning*
- *Took it easy at our apartment today*

23/06/15 10am Cycle Day 16 (day 1 for embryos)

- *Fertilisation results: 7 of the 8 eggs have fertilised – WOW! We are so thrilled! Hope our babies continue to grow and develop nicely and healthily.*
- *Slept in this morn as Bruce is sick and needed the sleep. He slept for 3 hours in the pram yesterday – he never does that.*
- *Feeling bloated and tender today, but pretty good really. Have to stop myself from doing too much. Going to get into some work – I am behind.*

24/06/15 Cycle Day 17 (day 2 for embryos)

Started Crinone (P₄) gel day and night

. . .

We were so happy that seven of the eight eggs fertilised = 87.5%! On their third day of life since fertilisation, when they should ideally be six to eight cells in size, we were informed we had four embryos at eight cells and three embryos at five cells in size (outside ideal range but still capable of catching up). Things were looking positive. I calculated our baby would be due 14/03/16.

Our week in Sydney was spent resting, watching movies, working, going for walks, enjoying different cuisines and catching up with old friends. Never far from our minds were our babies growing in their dishes at Genea. I wanted to support my body with acupuncture, so researched acupuncturists in the vicinity of where we were staying. I tried a few and was able to get in with a Chinese Herbalist and Acupuncturist named

Lily in Surry Hills who, from my limited research, had a special interest in fertility. "I'll give her a go," I thought. Visiting Lily's clinic was a very unique experience. She captivated me as she buzzed around giving all her energy to her clients who were tucked away in tiny treatment rooms all around the building. She was genuinely interested in my well-being and our IVF success. She was all about East meets West for better health, and it boosted my spirits. I truly appreciate being in the presence of passionate, skilled practitioners. On my first visit I walked out with A LOT of Chinese herbs and some cryptic handwritten instructions to start following right away.

Lily squeezed me in for a second appointment the day before our embryo transfer. Now being squeezed in to an already overflowing schedule means being prepared to wait for a very long time, hope you're not forgotten and make a dash for it as soon as someone gives you the signal you're up. I did eventually have an acupuncture treatment and from there ended up with two bags of Chinese ingredients to make Lily's extraordinary 'glue' recipe and Ginseng Chicken Soup. I had spent over $1,000 with her in two days, but her belief in her medicine and her fertility track record meant it was hard to walk out without it. I was willing to try anything. Adam wasn't so sure when I got back to our apartment, mind you! Lily told me to keep in close contact so we could modify the concoction of Chinese herbal medicine as I moved through the cycle.

Adam stayed at our apartment to take care of Bruce while I caught an Uber to Genea for the embryo transfer at 9am on Cycle Day 20. We were blessed to have a 'prime quality' hatching blastocyst to transfer five days after fertilisation. Another Day 5 embryo was placed on ice at the blastocyst stage, while all the others didn't make it to that stage. We were excited to have two frozen embryos for a later date, and hopefully never have to go through a stimulated IVF cycle again. We drove back to Gunnedah that day and I kept my lucky red merino socks on the entire time.

The twenty-eighth of June, one day post transfer, was a hugely special day for us. It was the day we would officially start the next chapter of life at our new farm "Horsley Park," hopefully as a family of four. Our embryo was where it should be, but was it going to successfully implant? I hoped with all my heart it was. I absolutely would not recommend one day post transfer driving four hours, stopping in Goondiwindi to pack the remainder of your belongings from your sister's house into two vehicles while minding Bruce, driving some more to arrive at your new home at 4:30pm to an utterly bare house except for the huge room on the end jam-packed full (like Tetris) to the ceiling with almost every item you own. And then from 4:30pm to 9pm attempt to set up a few basics in the house while Adam and your brother-in-law Anthony move furniture into position. I really pushed myself that day and was so worried I'd compromised our chance of implantation. The crazy things you do.

Although there was a whole house to set up, I forced myself to take it easier two and three days post transfer – for my own sake as well as Bruce's and our new little one's. My energy levels were low and I felt 'off,' but other than that I'd been feeling quite normal which I was analysing to the death. Shouldn't I be feeling more by now? Was it a good sign, bad sign or not a sign at all? "Come on little bubby, burrow in down there," I told him/her.

I was doing my daily meditation, taking Lily's herbs (which tasted disgusting) and I'd also found a big pot in a kitchen box to cook up Lily's Chinese 'glue' recipe (to glue the embryo in!), which I was to take along with my herbs. I felt like a witch cooking up the glue brew. It included some amazing ingredients, even deer antler, but unfortunately didn't taste amazing. Her herbal medicines seemed pretty potent and I was running with the theory that it could only help.

Adam and I were blissfully happy to be living at Horsley Park – a mixed farm on which we produced crops and beef cattle. It felt like home straight away. It was our dream come true. For the first time in months, we stopped and took a breath which was a nice change from the pressure we'd been under.

Four days post transfer I started to feel some intermittent feelings in my boobs, ovaries, abdomen and lower back. I tried not to focus on it and kept unpacking, catching up on Sunburnt Country work and getting sorted on the farm. This did trigger the question: how long will I last before I cave and do a home pregnancy test...?

By seven days post transfer I was experiencing some distinct symptoms that I could no longer ignore: bloating, shortness of breath, lethargy, frequent urination, cramping in lower back and also wind pain. I couldn't help myself... I did a pregnancy test... and it was a faint positive. BUT I couldn't rely on this because the Ovidrel (hCG) injection can stay in your system for 10-14 days and produce a false positive test. So, I had to contain myself.

The next day, eight days post transfer, another positive and slightly darker line on the test. And diarrhoea started.

Two days later ten days post transfer, another positive and even darker line. I couldn't believe it! Ad and I started to allow a glimmer of hope to enter our hearts. The diarrhoea and other symptoms continued. I was perplexed and (really not enjoying) the diarrhoea. What was causing it – the water at the farm? The Chinese herbs? Maybe a gastro bug?

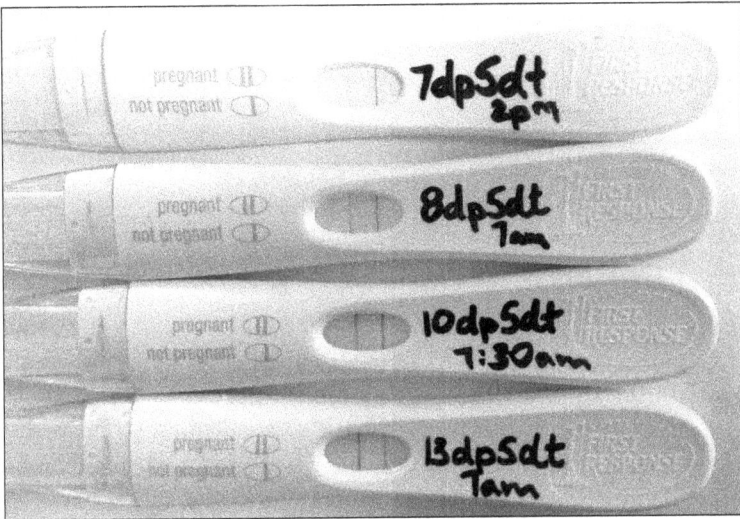

When one positive pregnancy test is never enough! "Horsley Park" July 2015.

I rang Rhonda eleven days post transfer to talk about the awful bloating and diarrhoea. She said it sounded like OHSS. Huh? It hadn't even crossed my mind that hyperstimulation could cause diarrhoea. The next morning was my scheduled pregnancy blood test so Dr. Livingstone included a full blood count to check my HCT. I was instructed to rest and drink lots of water. With the positive home pregnancy tests and possible OHSS, we were cautiously optimistic we'd have a favourable blood test result, but there was still that lingering fear.

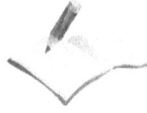

09/07/15 12 days post transfer

hCG = 510! ("gee that's high" said both Rhonda and Lily)

Progesterone = 200

Oestrogen = 2000

We're having a baby!! And the results show that I'm not hyper stimulated over the threshold! Can stop Crinone immediately. Diarrhoea is still going. Some dull cramps and feeling yukky with no energy.

Thank you, God for the miracles in my life – the one sleeping in his cot and the other growing inside me.

. . .

It was implausible that we had a positive result on another first cycle IVF attempt. It just seemed too good to be true and I kept fearing the worst. Surely, we couldn't be that lucky? Did we deserve this?

As the weeks went on, I continued to feel pretty darn awful and the diarrhoea continued intermittently (for nine weeks). At seven weeks pregnant, I looked 12 weeks. I suspected there was something more happening here. I had a sneaking suspicion I was carrying more than one little Benschicle. Was it as the tarot card reader predicted?

Before the sonographer had a chance to announce it, Adam and I spotted two little jelly beans on the screen at my seven week ultrasound. I whispered to him, "Did you see that? There's another one?" We shared a look that I'll never forget. A few minutes later the scan confirmed two little heartbeats. It was the most incredible sight to behold. I didn't know whether to laugh or cry, so I did a bit of both. Afterwards we wandered out of the building into the sunlight, stunned. Two babies! We had just entered a whole new world that was completely alien to us – twin land.

The sonographer's report stated that the twins were monochorionic monoamniotic which meant they were in the same gestational sac and sharing the same placenta – a very high risk pregnancy – so this was not encouraging news. I was devastated at the prospect of losing our babies. Thankfully, a few weeks later a scan revealed a membrane between the two which meant they were monochorionic diamniotic (MoDi twins) – sharing the same placenta but in individual sacs. It was still high risk but with less possible complications.

This result also meant they were identical twins. The odds of this are about one in 250 pregnancies, so it's not all that rare, but not all that common either. We had had only one embryo transferred, so we learned that the embryo must have randomly split between five and eight days after conception. Incredible. Maybe when I was lifting boxes and shouldn't have been?

If I thought IVF was challenging, there was a whole lot more challenging ahead. It was a stressful and intensively monitored pregnancy, but we were fortunate to get through it without any major health concerns for me or the babies.

Our identical blue-eyed, curly haired twin boys Bronson and Myles were born eight minutes apart on the eighteenth of February 2016 at 36 weeks and one day. How blessed we are is not lost on us for a second. Though it's difficult to tell them apart by looks, they couldn't be more different in personality, and have been since the beginning. To describe them a little: Bronson is independent, gentle and precise; Myles is creative, outgoing and sensitive.

Bruce celebrated his second birthday in the hospital common room with a supermarket-bought red velvet cake, while closely watching his tiny twin brothers ("the bubbas" as he calls them) in their hospital cot.

**For detailed medical notes from this IVF cycle please see the Appendix.

A special note about support

Even with the support of my closest friends and family, I've never felt as isolated and alone as I did going through fertility treatment in rural Australia. I drove for hours to appointments on my own, sat in waiting rooms for hours by myself, underwent procedures alone, with no one to talk to that would truly 'get it.' I didn't know where to access support other than through a counsellor or online IVF forums (I did a lot of that).

It was tough.

I could see the need for a local support group in Goondiwindi, and considered starting one, but then that would have put the spotlight on me, and would anyone join anyway? And how long would I need it for? Hopefully only briefly. Instead, I sent a virtual hug to envelope anyone in the community who was also going through what I was.

I had two friends having IVF through Genea around the same time as me and I had no clue. This demonstrated to me how silently and privately this battle is usually fought. One friend lived in the country – Susie,* and one lived in Sydney – Laura.*

During our 2015 IVF round, Susie and I literally nearly ran into each other at the ultrasound clinic in Tamworth where we were both having follicle tracking scans. We were then in Sydney over the same period for the remainder of our treatment cycles. In fact, our egg retrieval procedures were on the same morning and I saw Susie and her husband in recovery at Genea. I felt like a veteran, while it was her first time.

She was the first 'real' person I could talk to or swap notes with who was going through the same thing at the same time. But it didn't work out that way. It wasn't something that you wanted to swap notes on because there was far too much raw emotion involved and comparing as we went was not beneficial for either of us. That was an interesting learning: it was better to send general messages of support, but not talk specifics like the number of eggs retrieved, eggs fertilised or embryos to transfer. It was really nice to have an IVF buddy, but it was also awkward in some respects. She was very private, I was more open. I questioned what I should say and when, and decided sometimes less is more.

I was devastated to learn that Susie's treatment cycle was not successful and felt ashamed to report that ours was. It was hard to tell her our news and I experienced what it's like when the shoe is on the other foot. The guilt was crippling. Out of respect to her I wanted her to be one of the first to know, but I had to work up the courage because I knew it was going to hurt.

Laura was very private too and didn't wish to share many details other than that their embryo transfer didn't result in a pregnancy. I felt so sorry. Thankfully both she and Susie did eventually have success.

What I came to realise is that even when you have access to support (formal or informal), you may or may not use it. I was envious of the women having their morning blood tests and scans at the fertility clinics in the city while I drove for hours and sat on my own. I felt angry at times. However, I now know that I may have felt equally as alone sitting in the crowd. I also came to learn that even if I'd had a face-to-face support group available to me, I still could have isolated myself if I chose to – and that may have changed from one month to the next. Even though Susie, Laura and I were having the same treatment at the same time, our experiences were not the same.

We can isolate ourselves as little or as much as we choose regardless of our location. It's such an intensely personal, emotion-laden journey handled differently by every individual and couple.

In the wider community the conversation around TTC swings wildly. It can be a taboo topic and avoided completely, and in other spaces it's loosely thrown around in conversation like talking about what's on special at the supermarket. Very rarely does anyone actually *really* talk about it with genuine curiosity and concern though, which has astonished me. I've concluded that it makes the average person VERY uncomfortable to broach the subject, so they don't. No one wants to say the wrong thing. It's a painful topic to talk about… so they usually don't.

If you are supporting someone going through a challenging time trying to conceive, please seek to understand first. Increase your awareness on the topic and be compassionately curious. If they give you an opening to explore the topic, be sure to ask questions, to listen, not to reply. Really listen, let them talk. Some simple open-ended questions to get started may be:

How are you?

How can I support you?

What can I do to help?

Would you like to talk more about it?

Whatever you do, keep any judgement and sweeping comments to yourself. You don't need to have any answers or stories, there is no 'right' thing to say. The greatest gift you can give them is to listen and have an open heart.

Real names have been substituted for privacy.

CHAPTER 12

Trying to Move On

I always wanted four children. I don't know why exactly. Was it in my DNA to yearn for four offspring? Was it that I thought families with four kids were cool? Maybe because I am one of four and it feels normal to me? I love having three siblings – it's like we're our own mini gang. I feel like my brother and sisters are 'my people' and I am blessed that we are tight-knit. Whatever the reason, when I pictured our future children there were four of them.

Adam, on the other hand, was very content with three. When for a long time the idea of having one child seemed to us like the hardest thing in the universe to achieve, we didn't get carried away worrying about what our final head count would be. After my pregnancy with the twinkles (our nickname for the twins) and surviving the rough early days with twins and a toddler, the thought of having another got well and truly shelved for a while. That was until the twins were about six months old – in that cute, chubby stage when life begins to get fractionally easier – when I started to entertain the thought of another.

I commented to Adam in jest, "Maybe we should have another one, babe?"

He said, with a grin, "It's not happening, Benita," and that's where we left it. I didn't fully believe him, and at that point I didn't fully believe myself either. Did I *really* want another? Did I *really* want to go through the trying all over again? I was so sleep-deprived most of the time that I could barely decide what I was eating for lunch, so having a rational conversation on such a pivotal topic firstly with myself, and then with Adam, was not really sensible.

About once a month I raised the idea of having another baby. At first, I was semi-joking but as the months went by there was increasing sincerity and desire behind my words, and those conversations with Adam began to start with, "Babe, can I please talk to you about something?" (the question every man dreads).

I told him that I was finding it difficult to move past the feelings I had about wanting another baby, and then I would present to him all the reasons why we should. I said that we needed to make a decision soon because guess what, time was a-ticking. Even if it didn't happen naturally, we had our two snow babies waiting for us in Sydney. I could fly to Sydney on my own for a frozen embryo transfer and be back within a few days. I put to him that if we didn't succeed with the embryos we had then I would let this go. Deal? Buh-bow, no deal. Adam had made his decision.

He was very clear on all the practical reasons we shouldn't. None of the reasons were that he couldn't love another child – he absolutely could. He thought I should be happy with what I had right in front of me and to put my energy into our boys. We'd been through so much in the last six years to create them and bring them safely into this world, why go back down that path? He was so resilient, that at times I needed reminding he, too, had endured a lot. I think he'd had enough and was ready to get on with the next part of life.

I knew the suggestion sounded a bit crazy as it fell from my lips. I knew the risks, the what-ifs and the possibilities. I'd contemplated all of them. But I also knew the abundance of everything that we had to offer another child, and the blessing he or she would be to complete our family. I couldn't shake the vision in my mind of four little Bensch people.

"Right Benita, come on, chin up, he's right you know, it doesn't make sense to pursue this."

My thinking brain knew that everything he was telling me was logical. This is where it started to get tricky.

The truth was – I wasn't done. I just wasn't. The longing wouldn't go away. There was still a gap in my heart and a dream unfulfilled. Turns out that the maternal drive I once lacked was now so strong!

Or was I conjuring up this idea in my mind because for so long I'd wanted a baby and now I was permanently in this baby-creating phase and couldn't move on? Was I just too scared to get on with life? The debate raged on within me – a see saw of a different nature.

It was March 2017. For the best part of the last seven years, I'd been focused on thinking about, talking about, trying for, being pregnant with, and caring for babies. Why wasn't I content with three? Three is what the tarot card reader saw for us. Three was wonderful, three was plenty! Some people had none. Our sanity and marriage barely survived the first year with three children two years and under. Why would I jeopardise that by adding another into the chaos?

It was the first time in our relationship that Adam and I totally disagreed on something of significance. It was a new experience for us and not enjoyable for either party. There was more than a white elephant in the room, it was a huge, ugly, woolly, tusky mammoth. A pattern emerged: I would start the conversation, we'd end up in a fight, I would stew on it for a few days, talk myself out of the idea and then push it down. Then as the weeks went on it would rise up within me again.

Adam began to get very frustrated with me and he would say, "I'm not going to change my mind and I don't want to talk about it again." I didn't let it go because I thought I could sway him. I truly did. It enraged me that he could have the power to decide. Why did he get to make the decision? Why should he have it his way? I didn't like causing this friction between us; I tried to help him understand it was a feeling I couldn't easily dismiss.

The last discussion we had about it became heated and I lost it. All of the sorrow and the rage erupted in a torrent of yelling and tears. He wouldn't budge. At the end I walked away, defeated. I rang my Mum the next day to talk it through and we came up with all the arguments that backed what Adam was saying:

You've got three other children to consider – they have to come first.

What about your age?

What about the cost?

What if there are pregnancy complications?

What if there are health issues?

What about the toll on your body and bouncing back after the baby?

Can your marriage survive the pressure of another baby so soon?

Isn't it time to move on and concentrate on something else?

Exactly. Logic had to prevail, I told myself. It was either Adam or I who had to compromise and it looked like it was going to be me. After all, I couldn't win this battle without him.

It wasn't what I wanted in my heart, but I recognised I had to start accepting this reality and move on. Gently and slowly I began the process of letting go and allowing myself the luxury of questioning what came next: what do I want to do, who does post-baby Benita want to be? It was scary! The best way I knew to get past this was to apply myself to something to propel me forward. On top of nurturing our beautiful boys, it was time to get my business brain back in gear and focus on our agricultural business.

I delayed finishing breastfeeding the twins to relish that part of mother-hood for a little longer, as I knew now they would be my last babies. They had their last feed at bedtime on the twenty-eighth of May at just over 15 months old. I was sentimental, but I had made progress in the past few months and had gotten to a point of feeling more enthusiastic about what lay ahead. It was time to start a new chapter.

It turns out the universe had other plans…

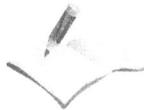

08/07/17

Years of heartache. Years of therapies and procedures. So many needles, drugs and scans. Tens of thousands of dollars. Tens of thousands of kilometres. That's what it took to bring our three precious little men into the world. We conceived naturally once (that we know of) in all that time (and lost the baby). And now here I sit, in total and utter disbelief, that yesterday I had a positive pregnancy test. WHAT.THE.HELL. How on Earth did that happen… all on its own… with no planning, no assistance, not even folic acid supplements for 3 months in the lead up to trying to conceive like the good book says. NOTHING. I simply cannot believe the irony of it. I used to genuinely struggle to understand how anyone, ANYONE, could simply 'discover' they were pregnant. Those people that could conceive in their first month of trying, or not trying at all, and they'd say 'it happened quicker than we thought.' And I'd think 'what the fuck?' Not only did I struggle with it, for a long time I wanted to give those people a fly kick to the head! Now I am one of them. And I feel so guilty! I feel like a traitor to the club I've belonged to for so long. I'm sorry everyone. I don't know how this happened (well actually I do know how this happened and I feel like an irresponsible, cheeky teenager). Secretly though, I am delighted. And a bit scared. And I am so bloody proud of us! We actually did it, all on our own! Wow. This little one was obviously meant to be, and has been making his/her way to us all these years. Dear Universe and God, please allow us to keep him/her and bring him/her into our lives safely. Thank you for the enormous blessing of four little people to love.

. . .

Mum warned me as a teenager, "If you play with fire, you're going to get burned." What a joke that seemed through all the years of TTC and in the end, there I sat, taking heed. Mum is always right in the end.

As it turned out, the date of conception was the nineteenth of June – my 36th birthday!

Within days of my birthday I had a very strong feeling I was pregnant. Two days on I Googled 'can you know you're pregnant two days after conceiving?' because I just *felt* pregnant. I had obviously had a bit of pregnancy experience to go on by this stage, but I still couldn't whole-heartedly trust the feeling that I was pregnant. I found myself having no ability to control my fingers that tapped 'early pregnancy symptoms' into the search box. Seriously, what *was* I doing? Old habits die hard.

The inner dialogue started. Mrs. O. and Mrs. R. came back to visit on their seesaw.

I was uncharacteristically reserved and didn't share my suspicions with Adam. Only after a week of feeling seething anger towards him (for no good reason) did I say to a friend when she visited for a coffee, "Maybe I'm pregnant?" Hearing those words out in the open and not just in my head breathed life into them.

As the due date of my period came closer, I had some physical PMT-ish symptoms that I hadn't been getting with my monthly period since the twins were born. This time there wasn't fertility drugs involved so I was able to distinguish what was being caused by my body versus the drugs. In fact, I wasn't even on the pill because I had stood firm that I was done with that, and any other hormonal drugs, for a good while (or ever).

The due date came and went and still nothing.

The night before I took a pregnancy test, Adam and I were sitting in the lounge room and I calmly said "Babe, I'm nearly certain that I'm pregnant." If only I had a dollar for the number of times I'd said that over the years! I'm pretty sure Ad was rolling his eyes in his mind thinking, "This woman… here we go again!"

He said, "You've thought that plenty of times before, and you weren't, so let's just see what happens." It was a touchy subject to bring up given our discussions over the previous six months, so I tried to deliver it with neutrality. I didn't tell him I was planning to do a test the next morning.

What I found confusing is that although Adam was saying he didn't want a fourth child, he wasn't exactly taking extra steps to be 'careful.' Something about it didn't add up, even when I cautioned him around the middle of the month that we should be more careful. It was a game. I was telling him we should be more careful, and secretly hoping I'd fall pregnant. He was playing with fire but saying he didn't want another. We felt like the chances of conceiving naturally were very slim given our history, but I think we were both secretly testing the hypothesis. We didn't admit it to each other at the time, but deep down we both wanted to prove we could achieve this on our own.

The next morning I slipped out of bed and did my usual pregnancy test routine with the associated mental torment that doesn't seem to abate no matter how many tests you do. It wasn't super early – our three sons were awake lying in our bed with Adam while he pretended he was asleep (hoping they might go back to sleep).

When the second pink line quickly appeared in the results window, I wasn't totally surprised. But that feeling… that indescribable feeling. Only a wall separated me from the boys, but in that moment I wasn't in the room, I was in heaven. I savoured it on my own in the bathroom for a moment.

Oh my God. Oh my God. Oh my God.

Is this how it can happen… so easily? To us?

We did it.

We did it…

We did it!

But gosh, what was Adam going to say?

I gathered myself and rounded the wall into the bedroom. Adam was lying on his left side facing away from me toward the boys who were huddled together on my side of the bed – a mass of three and one-year-old boyness.

"How do you feel about being a father of four?" I asked gently.

He turned his head to look at me, wide-eyed, gauging whether I was serious. I didn't know whether to smile or stay straight-faced. I honestly had no idea how he would react – whether he would be happy or fly out bed swearing! As he rolled back over murmuring something I didn't catch (there may have been an F-bomb in there), there was a cheeky Adam Bensch grin on his face. In that moment I knew we were going to be okay.

As we cooked breakfast, Ad was sprouting on about all the logistics:

"We'll have to get a new car…"

"There's no way we can afford boarding school for four kids…"

"How are we going to have enough land for all of them?"

I let him go while I practically sashayed around the kitchen with a foolish smile on my face, already dreaming of the little human growing inside me.

"We'll work it out, it will all be okay," I said.

With this pregnancy we became one of those stories you detest hearing when you're TTC that goes a bit like this, "My cousin's friend went through IVF six times and then they fell pregnant naturally." On a bad day I would think, "Whatever… good on them, that's fairy tale stuff, that's no help to me."

We were astounded that we got a fairy tale ending.

16/09/17 14w14d pregnant

I wonder if it was meant to be all along that we would experience what it's like to create a life all on our own. I wonder if it was always in our plan – for healing and for closure. And also to experience how it looks and feels on the other side. I almost feel apologetic when telling people about expecting #4. Why? Because I feel bad for everyone I've left in my old club. Like the beautiful friend who started trying at the same time as us seven years ago and still doesn't have a baby. Another beautiful friend that has one little boy after many rounds of IVF, but has not been able to have another.

. . .

We were overjoyed to welcome Lawson (aka Mr. Natural) into the world on his 40 week due date – the thirteenth of March 2018. He is the finest surprise we could ever have received into our family. With his blue eyes, curly blonde hair, and cheeky nature, he is a force to be reckoned with. He is also a cuddly little bear.

When women used to tell me they knew they were 'done' with having children, I wondered what that actually felt like. I wondered if I would ever feel it. I hoped that I would know when I was done. Now I do.

The clock has stopped ticking.

The trying is no more.

CHAPTER 13

Trying with a positive mental attitude

WITH GUEST AUTHOR KAREN BROOK

The importance of developing and maintaining a positive attitude became more evident, and challenging, as our TTC journey continued. As you've learned, I went to some dark places along the way. It wasn't until I started to take deliberate daily action such as guided meditation, reciting affirmations and the work I was doing on myself through my coaching study, that I felt more empowered and in control of myself. I still had down and negative moments, or days (which is okay and normal), but overall I was in a healthier state in mind, body and spirit to conceive.

This chapter is written by a successful mentor of mine, Karen Brook. Through my work with Karen, I am continually developing my mind to create the results I want in my life. I highly recommend you absorb what she has written, and more importantly: do what she says! I wish that when we were TTC I had had this awareness and the tools she offers here.

How to develop a positive mental attitude

BY KAREN BROOK

I'm sure you've had many people tell you to keep a "positive attitude" and it will happen, right? Well, what does that mean anyway? Most people who talk about attitude have absolutely no idea what it really means. You can be an outwardly positive person, but still be thinking thoughts of lack or limitation and not feel so good, despite what you project to the outside world.

One of the best things you can do to support yourself in falling pregnant and experiencing a happy, healthy pregnancy is to develop a positive mental attitude. Your attitude is the composite of your thoughts, feelings and actions expressed. It's an energy you send off into the universe and it dictates what you attract back. You want to be putting your mind and body in the most relaxed, beautiful state and be in control of it as you walk your conception to parenthood journey.

Let's break this down further and put you to work. Take out a notepad and pen and outline your current attitude as it stands today:

Thoughts: *What thoughts have you been having about your current situation or the results you've been receiving?*

Feelings: *How have these thoughts been making you feel?*

Actions: *What actions are you taking or not taking based on these thoughts and feelings? How are your thoughts and feelings influencing your behaviour on a day-to-day basis?*

Now think about the result or the outcome that you want to accomplish. For example, imagine you are now carrying a healthy baby and experiencing a great pregnancy. Even go one step further to imagine that you now have a thriving six-week-old baby and you're loving being a Mum!

What would your new thoughts, feelings and actions be? Imagine yourself there. What kind of attitude would you have?

Thoughts: *How am I thinking now that I am observing and experiencing the results I really want?*

Feelings: *How are these thoughts making me feel? E.g. Calm, content, happy, joyous*

Actions: *Now that I am thinking and feeling like this, what actions am I taking day-to-day? Is this behaviour in line with what I want?*

It's important to bring your attitude – your thoughts, feelings and actions – into alignment with the results you want. You must express one clear vibration (of energy) of your desire to bring you in harmony with what you want. You don't get what you want, you get who you are and are willing to become.

Write out your new attitude at least once a day, every day for the next 30 days. Carry it with you, read it as often as you can, and move into action with the new actions and behaviours now even though it may feel uncomfortable. You must act as if you are already there. Do the things you'd do if you were already experiencing a healthy pregnancy or have your little ones at your feet. It might sound a bit 'out there' and feel risky, but it works.

The proper use of your imagination

The truth is that you are God's/Universe's highest form of creation and you have a power flowing to and through you that will take any idea you turn over to it and begin at once to move it into physical form. Your imagination is one of six mental faculties you have at your aid to help you create what you want. The creative principle is always on the inside and the outside is always a reflection of what's happening on the inside.

Your imagination is your real self. Your imagination will take you anywhere you want to go. As far as your subconscious mind is concerned, any idea or emotion experienced in imagination is real. Your subconscious mind cannot tell the difference between what is real and what is imagined. So, as you begin to imagine yourself already in possession of what you want and allow yourself to experience the emotions and feelings that go with that, your subconscious mind accepts it as truth. This has an immediate effect on how you feel in your body and ultimately your behaviour and results.

Let's build a beautiful, crystal clear picture of what you want and see yourself as already having it.

Close your eyes and totally relax. Let a beautiful picture of your desire form on the screen of your mind (imagination) and see the picture through your own eyes. You are one with it and it is one with you. What do you see, how does it feel? What are you doing? Really allow yourself to get into this without judging or blocking what you're seeing.

Take some time to write out the picture in the present tense and with positive language. Start your writing with *I am so happy and grateful now that...*

It's important for you to form the discipline of seeing yourself where you want to be and then be there. You will need to practise this many times and keep doing it every day until it becomes habit. Train yourself in the deliberate use of your imagination so you can stay focused and connected to what you want, rather than being focused on the present circumstances and results. Your current reality is not your point of support - your point of support is always inside.

Tapping into the power of gratitude

Wallace D. Wattles in *The Science of Getting Rich* has this to say about the power of gratitude, "The whole process of mental attunement and atonement can be summed up in one word: GRATITUDE."

Gratitude will lead you out of the darkness and into the light. A grateful mind will keep you in closer touch with the source from which good things flow and will keep you from being displeased with your present results or current reality.

The following daily practice of gratitude was taught to me by my mentor, Bob Proctor. Now I am passing it onto you.

It's a three-step exercise:

1. Reflect on and write down 10 things you feel truly grateful for. This can be past results, present results and also results manifesting in your future – like your goal of a healthy baby. Give gratitude everyday by writing, "I am so happy and grateful now that I have a healthy, happy baby," or "I am so happy and grateful now that I am experiencing a perfectly healthy pregnancy," or "I am so happy and grateful now that I am at my ideal pregnancy weight."

2. Sit quietly for five minutes and ask for guidance from God/Source for the day ahead. Notice any thoughts or ideas you get during this time and as you go about your day. You have a built-in guidance system that will help you get where you want to go. Trust it. It knows the path to your goal and what you want.

3. Send love to those who bother you. Someone once told me when you hate on another person, it's like you're drinking poison and hoping the other person dies. Let it go. Maybe you even need to send some love to yourself.

If you would like a complimentary gratitude pad to go with this exercise, write to me at karen@karenbrook.com.au and I'd be happy to send you one. It's such a powerful habit to develop and it will change your life.

In closing **I want you to remember that you are in control**. As you gain and take control from within, you bring order and calmness to the world around you. Focus on a positive mental attitude despite the circumstances by choosing thoughts, feelings and actions that are in harmony with what you want (rather than present results). Use your imagination daily to move you to the place you want to be, and use the practice of gratitude to keep you connected to the source from which greater good flows.

––––––––

Karen Brook is an entrepreneurial expert, a results mentor and someone who is passionately focused on converting thinking into results. Karen works closely with individuals and teams helping them be the best at what they do and multiply their influence, impact and income in life, business and careers through teaching internationally acclaimed Bob Proctor's proven methodologies. She is the No.1 consultant in the world facilitating Bob Proctor's proven methodology for success known as "Thinking Into Results." Based in Brisbane, she has built a global community of "thinkers and doers" who are co-creating together to help each other accomplish tremendous goals in their own lives. To learn more and connect with Karen visit www.karenbrook.com.au or find her on social media @karenbrook.

CHAPTER 14

My gift to you: Affirmations

An affirmation is a short, positive, present-tense, high-impact statement than can have a profound effect when impressed on the subconscious through repetition. Like me, I'm sure you've heard of affirmations, but you may not have used them effectively in your life to date. Essentially what you are doing with an affirmation is creating a positive thought that flows on to your feelings, actions and ultimately your results.

I (accidentally) discovered pregnancy affirmations the day before the embryo transfer in our first round of IVF and it was a revelation to me that I could use them to help me in my quest. I had a beautiful feeling wash over me when I started to read them, so I continued to do so on a regular basis even though I didn't understand what was happening in my mind.

I have crafted this selection of affirmations for you to use on your journey to parenthood. I hope you find the power in them that I have. I understand that affirmations alone will not get you pregnant, but they will absolutely support you through the process. I suggest you create your own affirmations to add to these.

How to use these affirmations

1. Choose and focus on one or two affirmations at a time that resonate with you. Get involved in the repetition of them for a period of time such as 30 days, and then you can change or add another one or two. This will begin to change your subconscious beliefs about the whole pregnancy journey and all the elements involved.

2. Repetition is critical! Read, say and write your affirmation as often as you can (at least once daily). Put it where you'll read it often, make a recording of it on your phone and play it on a loop. Be sure to write it out daily. This is key, particularly so if the affirmation is not in line with your subconscious programming and you feel sceptical or negative in any way as you read it. Impressing the affirmation over and over on the subconscious fixes it in the mind and only then will you create the results you really want. Commit to making it a habit as part of your daily routine.

3. Read your affirmation with as much belief and emotion as you can. Feel the feeling (joy, relief, happiness, love, etc) NOW that you are already in possession of what you want. As you read, say and write the affirmation, use your imagination to create a picture in your mind and tap into the feeling of it.

AFFIRMATIONS

I am so happy and grateful now that my body is ready right now to receive and nourish a baby.

I am so happy and grateful now that I trust everything is happening exactly as it should.

I am so happy and grateful now that I let everything in my life flow freely and easily. I only focus on those things that serve me toward my greater good.

I am so happy and grateful now that I am growing a healthy baby inside me.

I am so happy and grateful now that I trust in my body to create life.

I am so happy and grateful now that I conceive with ease.

I am so happy and grateful now that I am a mother.

I am so happy and grateful now that I am pregnant.

I am so happy and grateful now that I am calm and in control of my thoughts.

I am so happy and grateful now that I choose to accept only helpful thoughts.

I am so happy and grateful now that I am strong, safe and supported.

I am so happy and grateful now that I nourish my mind and body for optimum fertility.

I am so happy and grateful now that I use my positive mental attitude to create what I want in my life.

I am so happy and grateful now that I let go of what is outside my control.

I am so happy and grateful now that I let go of anything that no longer serves me.

I am so happy and grateful now that I have the gift of a child in my life.

I am so happy and grateful now that I have a healthy baby in my arms.

I am so happy and grateful now that I am experiencing a perfectly healthy pregnancy.

I am so happy and grateful now that I love my baby.

I am so happy and grateful now that my baby loves me.

I am so happy and grateful now that I welcome the changes in my body.

I am so happy and grateful now that I've created life.

I am so happy and grateful now that my body is perfect.

I am so happy and grateful now that my pregnant body is beautiful.

I am so happy and grateful now that my baby and I are healthy and strong.

I am so happy and grateful now that this is our time to conceive.

I am so happy and grateful now that my eggs are becoming perfectly healthy babies.

I am so happy and grateful now that I have a new month for new beginnings.

I am so happy and grateful now that I have all the courage I need in this moment.

I am so happy and grateful now that I allow a baby into my life.

I am so happy and grateful now that I am surrounded by support.

AFTERWORD

Adam and I are amongst the lucky ones. We got a happy ending, an overwhelmingly happy ending! We are grateful for our boys every single day and when I look at them, I wonder how we got to be so fortunate. Not everyone gets that opportunity and my heart aches for those who don't.

I have wondered a lot why we could only conceive naturally twice in seven years. Was it my endometriosis? My age? Something wrong with my eggs or ovulation? Stress? My hormone levels? Did I create the issue? Was it that I expected to have trouble falling pregnant and that is what came to be? I'd love to know the answers, but never will. I have nothing to back it up but I suspect it was a combination of factors. I now know I could have been so much more effective with my mindset to help us conceive – I wish I had known then what I know now in regards to harnessing the power of my mind.

Were we trying too much? What about if we'd been more patient and let nature take its course over time – would we have ended up with four children? I don't know. At the time I wished we didn't have to go through what we did, but I am thankful for it now. It taught me a lot about many things – the gift of human life; my incredible body; the role of complementary therapies; the wonder of modern science, technology and medicine; my magnificent mind; the resilience I didn't know I had; the power of human nature; the most important people in my life; and the strength of my relationship with Adam. I believe there was a lesson for me in who I had to become in order to receive our children.

Until recently I had the Circle + Bloom IUI + IVF meditations still stored in the music library of my mobile phone. Occasionally one would randomly play if I had my music playing on shuffle. It stopped me in my tracks and I was instantaneously transported back in time to those days with those feelings of anticipation, hoping, wondering and the elusive balance between staying positive whilst not getting my hopes up. It's those encounters that remind me just how colossal TTC was in my life.

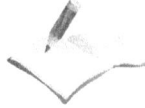

04/10/17

I am having a surreal moment. I am typing up the journal entries from our 2nd IVF cycle, with my mind and heart being transported back to that time and place, whilst watching the outcome of that cycle – our 19-month-old twin boys – play on the deck. Such a contradiction of emotions. I can feel the anguish of that past time course through my body, at the same time as feeling the joy of watching our beautiful children – here and in the flesh. The difficulty of that time still feels so real and not to be downplayed, but going through all of it was more than worth it.

. . .

There is one last piece of the story that knocked my socks off that I must share. When I asked Adam in September 2019 how he felt when I declared I was pregnant with Lawson, he replied that he was "happy" and he "wasn't surprised." Then, with a sneaky smile, he admitted to me for the first time ever that the idea of having #4 baby had "grown on him." All that anguish he put me through and it turns out in the end it's what he wanted as well! I knew it!

Here's a fun fact:

Bruce was conceived via IVF on the twenty-fifth of June 2013.

Bronson and Myles were conceived via IVF on the twenty-second of June 2015.

Lawson was conceived naturally on the nineteenth of June 2017.

People who don't know our story often say to me, "Gee, you planned that well! I know what you must have been doing on that same weekend every two years… wink, wink." Or they say, "Don't you have a TV, don't you know what causes that?" I chuckle to myself and think – "If only you knew!"

This year, 2019, we finally had my eternity ring made which, set in its band, has one diamond for each of our precious boys, and a glimmering emerald stone in honour of Ronnie Bean and the babies we have lost. Now I have them all with me all of the time.

It's an honour and a privilege to be a Mum, and to share my story with you. Thank you for reading. My greatest wish for you is: a fertile mind, body and spirit, and of course, babies! Wherever you are on your journey I send you my love, strength and best wishes. Please reach out if you need support.

With all my love,

Benita x

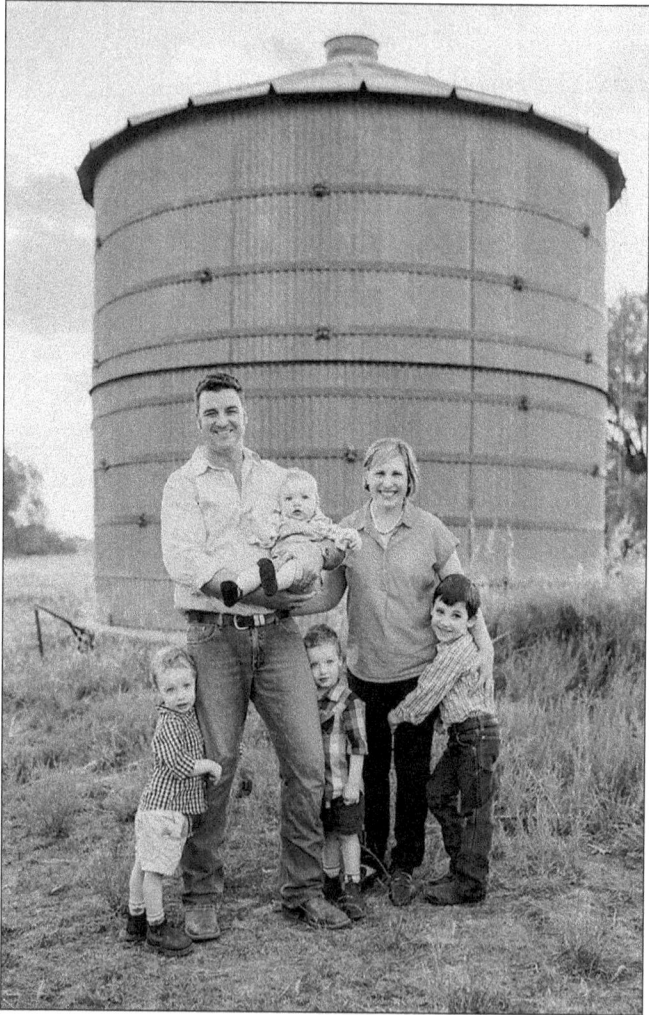

We did it. So incredibly blessed. Grong Grong December 2018.
Photo: Tegan Wilesmith, Sweet Lola Photography.

APPENDIX

Abbreviations

2WW	Two week wait
AI	Artificial insemination
AMH	Anti-Mullerial hormone
bhCG	beta human chorionic gonadotropin
BT	Blood test
E2	Oestradiol
FSH	Follicle stimulating hormone
GP	General Practitioner
hCG	Human chorionic gonadotropin
HCT	Haematocrit
ICSI	Intracytoplasmic sperm injection
IUI	Intrauterine insemination
IVF	In vitro fertilisation
LH	Luteinising hormone
NSW	New South Wales
OHSS	Ovarian hyper stimulation syndrome
OI	Ovulation induction
P_4	Progesterone
PMT	Pre-menstrual tension
Qld	Queensland
TTC	Trying to conceive

THE MEDICAL STUFF

The following medical summary is recorded to the best of my ability based on my records. **This does not constitute medical advice and it may not be a 100% complete record.**

13th February 2007

- Diagnostic laparoscopy and hysteroscopy performed to exclude any intrauterine abnormalities or the possibility of endometriosis. Also, cautery of the cervix.

- Mild-moderate endometriosis diagnosed. All visible lesions removed via diathermy. From report: "*Uterus normal and both adnexae tubes and ovaries normal, but Benita has endometriosis. A few clear lesions were seen in the anterior pouch to the right side and a few powder burn lesions in the Pouch of Douglas as well as on the left uterosacral ligament in the close vicinity of the left ureter as well as uterine artery.*"

- Adhesions also present. From report: "*Liver and vessels normal. There were some adhesions between the ascending colon to the right lateral abdominal wall and some congenital sigmoid adhesions to the left sidewall in the vicinity of the left adnexa.*"

- Cervical diathermy of ectropion performed.

20th November 2011

- Miscarriage at approximately 5.5 weeks gestation. Dilation and curettage not required.

January 2012

- Started Clomid 26th January 2012. Used for 1 cycle only.

September-December 2012

- 3 consecutive cycles of Ovulation Induction and Intrauterine Insemination. FSH injection dosage = Puregon 50.
  Ovulation trigger = Ovidrel 250.
  Luteal phase support = 2 progesterone pessaries/day.

Table 1. OI/IUI Cycle Monitoring Results.

Cycle day	Cycle 1 Monitoring		Cycle 2 Monitoring		Cycle 3 Monitoring	
	BT	Scan	BT	Scan	BT	Scan
7			E2 = 221 LH = 2 P4 = <1			
8	E2 = 387 LH = 1.8 P4 = <1					
9					E2 = 389 LH = 2.9 P4 = <1	
10			E2 = 683 LH = 2 P4 = <	Left = few @ 7mm Rt = 17mm, 3 approx. 13mm		
11	E2 = 250 (?) LH = 1 P4 = <1	Left = 12mm, 14mm, 16mm	E2 = 782 LH = 3.4 P4 = ?		E2 = 662 LH = 2.5 P4 = 0.6	Left = 7mm, 4 approx. 6mm Rt = 10mm, two approx. 6mm
12						
13	E2 = over 800	One follicle 20mm			E2 = 1080 LH = 5.4 P4 = 1.0	
14			Insemination			
15		Insemination				
16					E2 = 187 LH = 4.5 P4 = 6.9	

continued on next page

Cycle day	Cycle 1 Monitoring		Cycle 2 Monitoring		Cycle 3 Monitoring	
	BT	Scan	BT	Scan	BT	Scan
+7 (7dpo)	E2 = 387 P4 = 83.5		E2 = 419 P4 = 81.6			
+8 (8dpo)					E2 = 535 P4 = 25	
+9 (9dpo)						
+10 (10dpo)			P4 = 28 hCG = <5		P4 = 28.2 hCG = <5	
+11 (11dpo)						
+12 (12dpo)	P4 = 24 hCG = <5		P4 = 26 hCG = <5			
+13 (13dpo)						
+14 (14dpo)	P4 = 19 hCG = 0		Didn't record			

BT = Blood test, E2 = Oestradiol, LH = Luteinising Hormone, P4 = Progesterone, hCG = Human Chorionic Gonadotropin. Scan results = Follicular counts per ovary, dpo = days past ovulation.

13th March 2013

- Laparoscopy and hysteroscopy, dye through tubes, biopsy. Mild endometriosis found and cauterised.

June 2013

- Stimulated IVF cycle. FSH injection = Puregon 200. Antagonist = Orgalutran 250. Ovulation trigger = Ovidrel 250. Luteal phase support = Crinone 90mg (8%) gel twice/day.

Table 2. IVF Cycle 1 Monitoring Results.

Treatment Day (with FSH injections)	IVF Cycle 1 Monitoring	
	BT	Scan (Follicular Counts)
-1	E2 = 86	
1		
2		
3		
4	E2 = 352	
5		
6		
7		
8	E2 = 1127	Left = 12mm, two 14mm, 15mm Right = two <2mm, 12mm, two 14mm, 15mm, 16mm, 17mm
9		
10	E2 = 2273	
11		
12	Egg Retrieval	
13		
14		
15		
16		
17	E2 = 3408	
18	Embryo Transfer	
19 (1dpt)		
20 (2dpt)		
21 (3dpt)		
22 (4dpt)		
23 (5dpt)	E2 = 2890	
24 (6dpt)		
25 (7dpt)		
26 (8dpt)		
27 (9dpt)		
28 (10dpt)	E2 = 3240 hCG = 223	

BT = Blood test, E2 = Oestradiol, LH = Luteinising Hormone, P4 = Progesterone, hCG = Human Chorionic Gonadotropin. Scan results = Follicular counts per ovary, dpt = days post transfer.

- Egg retrieval: 10 eggs retrieved. One potentially immature. 10 eggs exposed to sperm. 80% fertilised = 8 fertilised eggs.
- Embryo development:

    Day 3 for embryos: (ideal is for embryos to be 6-8 cells)

    1 egg arrested after day 1 = 7 fertilised eggs left

    2x embryos 4 cells (likely not to develop any further)

    2x embryos 6 cells

    2x embryos 7 cells

    1x embryo 8 cells

    Day 5 for embryos:

    1x Grade 1 embryo transferred

    1x Grade 2 embryo frozen for future use
- Mild ovarian hyper stimulation syndrome.

June 2015

- Stimulated IVF cycle. FSH injection = Gonal-F 200. Antagonist = Orgalutran 250. Ovulation trigger = Ovidrel 250. Luteal phase support = Crinone 90mg (8%) gel twice/day.

Table 3. IVF Cycle 2 Monitoring Results.

Treatment Day (with FSH injections)	IVF Cycle 2 Monitoring	
	BT	Scan (Follicular Counts)
-1	E2 = 289 LH = 1.1 P4 = 1	
1		
2		
3		
4	E2 = 140	
5		
6		
7		
8	E2 = 753	Left = 10mm Right = two 10mm, 12mm, 15mm
9		
10	E2 = 1445	Left = 10mm, 15mm Right = five 12mm, 16mm, 20mm
11		
12	E2 = 2350	Left = 18mm, 22mm Right = 10mm, 12mm, 15mm, 16mm, 18mm, 19mm, 21mm, 22mm, 24mm
13		
14		
15	Egg Retrieval	
16		
17		
18		
19		
20	Embryo Transfer	
21 (1dpt)		
22 (2dpt)		
23 (3dpt)		
24 (4dpt)		

continued on next page

Treatment Day (with FSH injections)	IVF Cycle 2 Monitoring	
	BT	Scan (Follicular Counts)
25 (5dpt)		
26 (6dpt)		
27 (7dpt)		
28 (8dpt)		
29 (9dpt)		
30 (10dpt)		
31 (11dpt)		
32 (12dpt)	E2 = 2140, hCG = 510	

BT = Blood test, E2 = Oestradiol, LH = Luteinising Hormone, P4 = Progesterone, hCG = Human Chorionic Gonadotropin. Scan results = Follicular counts per ovary, dpt = days post transfer.

- Egg retrieval: 8 eggs retrieved. 8 eggs exposed to sperm. 87.5% fertilised = 7 fertilised eggs.
- Embryo development:

  Day 3 for embryos: (ideal is for embryos to be 6-8 cells)

  4x embryos 8 cells

  3x embryos 5 cells (still capable of catching up)

  Day 5 for embryos:

  1x Grade 1 embryo transferred

  1x embryo frozen for future use
- Suspected mild ovarian hyper stimulation syndrome.

ACKNOWLEDGEMENTS

Adam is the first and most important person in my life to acknowledge. Since we've been a couple we have been stretched, and stretched some more, in ways we never imagined. Your strength, stoicism and capacity for expansion while staying true to yourself continues to astound me. Your love for me regardless of the circumstances also astounds me, when I know I make life complicated! Thank you for your unrelenting belief in me and for allowing me to let our private story make its way to where it's needed. Thank you for supporting my dreams while being an incredible man and father. *As we grow together, I will walk with you wherever life may lead us and whatever may come.* I love you.

To Bruce, Bronson, Myles and Lawson:

I hope that by reading this story you will know how desperately Dad and I wanted you.

I hope that it will help you to know me not only as your Mum, but as a woman who fought to bring you into this world.

I hope that by capturing this story in words, you'll know a defining chapter of my life in which Dad and I grew – individually and as a team.

I hope you forgive me for taking the liberty of sharing the story of your creation before you are old enough to really understand.

I hope you know that regardless of how you were created, you are each unique and precious gifts – to me, to Dad and to the world.

I love you so much.

Mum and Dad, Kylee and Anthony, Shawn and Riana, Terri and John, Grandma and Pop Davis – you have supported me through everything, and you still do. What would I do without you? Thank you for pushing me to greater heights and reminding me who I am when I get a bit lost. Love you all.

To all the Bensch family – thank you for accepting me warts and all into your family, and for backing Adam and I to pursue our goals. Thank you for your love and support. I am blessed to have you in my life.

I have many special friends who have supported me through the good and the bad, and I am so thankful for you in my life. I would like to make particular mention of Mandy and Brody who have gone far above and beyond as friends to physically and emotionally help us through all the different stages we've been through. We are indebted to you guys. Thank you, we love you!

He'll say he was just doing his job, but I want to recognise Dr. Mark Livingstone for his excellence and his care, and for overseeing the medical content in this book. We were just another couple on his list of patients, but we never felt that way.

I'd like to thank Dr. Anna Carswell for her important contribution to this book as a medical practitioner, along with her ongoing medical care of our family.

To Judy, Anne, Corinne and the rest of the incredible team at Hasmark Publishing – thank you all! You were exceptionally patient and encouraging as you guided me through the publishing process. Your expertise was evident though you gently allowed me to lead the way to stay true to my vision.

A huge thanks to Jo of Jo Shanahan Photography for your energy, creative input and skill to capture the front cover photograph. It's been a pleasure working with you old friend.

Han McNulty of Dalli Photography – thank you for your generosity, your eye and skill in taking the photograph of me for the back, among others. You are an inspiration to me.

Thank you, Karen Brook for your insightful contribution to this book, for believing in me and holding a vision for me that I couldn't see for myself. I am so grateful to have your mentorship and your gentle nudging to give birth to this book and get it out into the world!

I'd like to thank Robert Gerrish who was the first to nurture my idea of writing this book. At that time my story wasn't complete, but the seed was planted and seven years later it's time for the harvest.

I would like to acknowledge all of the medical professionals whom I encountered on this journey that played their part in preparing me in mind and body to receive our children.

And lastly thank you to everyone who has encouraged me along the way during the writing and production of *The Art of Trying*. I really, truly appreciate it.

ABOUT THE AUTHOR

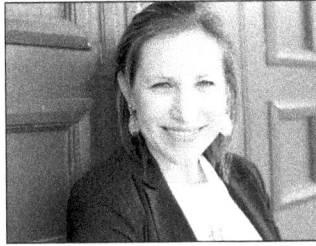

Photo: Hannah McNulty

Benita Bensch and her family own and operate a mixed farm near Moonie in south west Queensland, Australia, where Benita spreads her time among her family, writing, community and managing their farm and businesses with her husband Adam.

Benita holds a Bachelor of Rural Science (1st Class Hons), a Graduate Diploma in Business Studies (Marketing and Management) and her professional experience encompasses beef cattle genetics and extension, business management, public relations, marketing, project management, events and coaching.

Before children, Benita ran a successful small business specialising in marketing communications, branding and later, coaching. She is an experienced writer and accomplished speaker, having presented at numerous regional, state and national events on the topics of marketing, branding, business and personal development. In 2014 Benita was named in the Top 100 Women in Australian Agribusiness.

She loves being a Mum to four boys, running, planning, breeding Charolais cattle, getting up before the sun does, cooking, being of service to other women, being at home and the smell of rain.

This is her first book.

RESOURCES

These are sources I referred to or became aware of on my TTC journey. If you are outside Australia, you can simply do an internet search on the same subjects in your country.

Endometriosis Support

Endometriosis Australia: www.endometriosisaustralia.org

EndoActive: www.endoactive.org.au

Fertility Support

Genea: www.genea.com.au

AccessAustralia: www.access.org.au

Fertility Support: www.fertilitysupport.org.au

Miscarriage Support

SANDS: www.sands.org.au

Pregnancy Loss Australia: www.pregnancylossaustralia.org.au

The Pink Elephants Support Network: www.miscarriagesupport.org.au

Mental Health Support

Beyond Blue Support Service: www.beyondblue.org.au

SANE Australia: www.sane.org

Lifeline Australia: www.lifeline.org.au

Black Dog Institute: www.blackdoginstitute.org.au

CONNECT WITH BENITA

I invite you to connect with me personally so I can provide more value and assistance to you over time. Here's how you can:

Web: **www.benitabensch.com**
(I have an exclusive gift just for you, which you can access at www.benitabensch.com/extra)

Instagram: **@benitabensch**

Facebook: **@benitabensch**
I invite you to become a member of *The Art of Trying* community by joining *The Art of Trying* private Facebook group.

With love,

Benita x

BENITA BENSCH

HEARTS to be HEARD

Giving a Voice to Creativity!

Wouldn't you love to help the physically, spiritually,
and mentally challenged?

Would you like to make a difference
in a child's life?

Imagine giving them:
confidence; self-esteem; pride; and self-respect.
Perhaps a legacy that lives on.

You see, that's what we do.
We give a voice to the creativity in their hearts,
for those who would otherwise not be heard.

Join us by going to

HeartstobeHeard.com

Help us, help others.

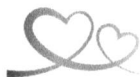